Follow Who Know Road: The path to Grow your Business as Licensed Insurance Producers/Agents

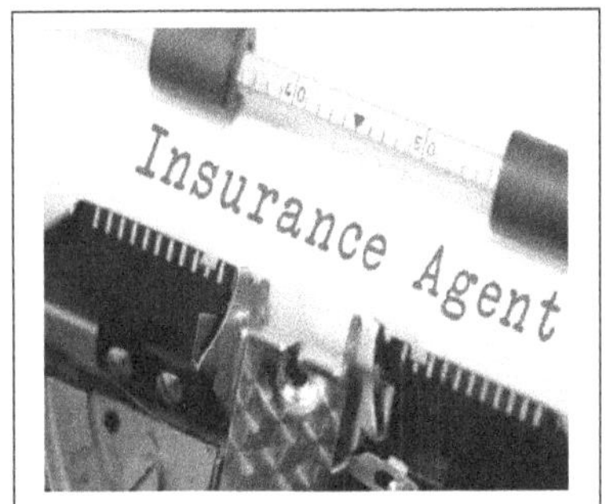

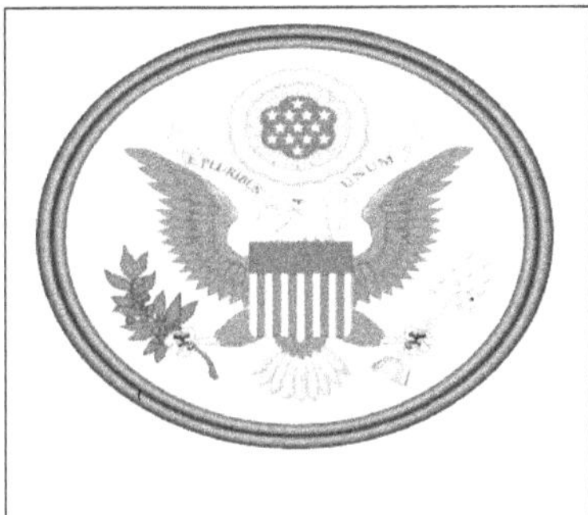

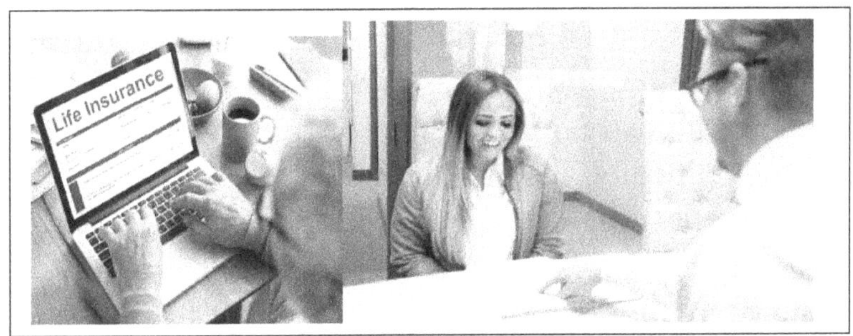

Dr. Joseph Gbanabom Conteh

Preface

In today's economic instability and hiking inflation, financial security has become more important than ever, the role of licensed insurance producers and agents stands out as one of purpose and impact. Yet, the path to success in this field is rarely straightforward. It requires more than product knowledge; it demands vision, strategy, discipline, and the willingness to learn from those who have already traveled the road to success. That is the essence of *Follow Who Know Road: The Path to Grow Your Business as Licensed Insurance Producers/Agents.*

This book is born out of a deep understanding of the challenges and opportunities in the financial and insurance industry. It is a guide for those who aspire to rise above mediocrity and build thriving careers while making a meaningful difference in their clients' lives. Whether you are a seasoned professional looking to refine your approach or a newcomer eager to find your footing, this book will serve as your trusted companion.

The title, *Follow Who Know Road*, is inspired by a timeless adage that highlights the importance of mentorship and learning from those with experience. It reflects the core message of this book: success leaves clues, and the fastest way to achieve your goals is by following in the footsteps of those who have already paved the way.

Each chapter is structured to answer fundamental questions:

Why? Discover your purpose and the driving force behind your career.

What? Define your vision, mission, goals, and objectives.

How? Learn actionable strategies to achieve success and navigate challenges.

Who? Understand the value of mentorship and the importance of being coachable.

Where? Identify the resources available to grow your business.

When? Commit your time and energy to consistent growth and improvement.

As you journey through these pages, you will find not just knowledge but inspiration and a roadmap to building a successful and fulfilling career. This is a call to action for professionals who are ready to take ownership of their growth, invest in themselves, and become part of a legacy of excellence in the financial services industry.

The path is clear. The tools are within reach. All that remains is your decision to act.

Let's begin this journey together. Follow who know road—and discover the limitless possibilities that await.

Dr. Joseph G. Conteh

Acknowledgements

I owe the creation of *Follow Who Know Road: The Path to Grow Your Business as Licensed Insurance Producers/Agents* to the remarkable individuals who have shaped my journey in this industry. This book is not just a guide; it is a tribute to the mentors and leaders who exemplify the values of excellence, care, and selflessness, inspiring me and countless others to rise above challenges and embrace opportunities.

To **Lylian Apono Akoh**, your daily gospel sermon, "Follow Who Know Road," has been a beacon of inspiration, motivating team members to persevere and thrive. Your unwavering dedication to uplifting others, combined with your love and care for their success, has left an indelible mark on our lives and communities. You are a leader in every sense, whose teachings resonate far beyond our industry and into the hearts of everyone fortunate enough to know you.

To **Mr. Fidelis Akoh**, your golden heart mirrors that of your angelic wife. Together, you are a force of nature, lifting "hungry souls" out of economic uncertainty and guiding them toward stability and success. Your kindness, humility, and commitment to building others up are a true testament to what it means to live with purpose.

To **Daniel Fombo and Angella Awudu**, your expertise, patience, and tireless commitment to developing and promoting strong, dynamic teams have created ripples of impact that will be felt for generations. You embody the principles of mentorship, proving that success is most rewarding when shared.

To every member of **Team Legacy** and **Team Optimum**, your collective passion and dedication have brought everlasting light into my soul and countless others. Your achievements are more than professional milestones; they are blessings to a world in need. Together, you have demonstrated that when people work with purpose and unity, they can transform lives and bring hope where it is most needed.

This book is a reflection of your guidance, your compassion, and the unparalleled example you have set. It is my honor to carry forward the lessons you have taught me, and I dedicate this work to you and to everyone who dares to dream, follow, and succeed.

With deepest gratitude,
Joseph Gbanabom Conteh

Dedication

This book is lovingly dedicated to **Angela Awudu, Lylian Apono Akoh, Fidelis Akoh, Daniel Fombo**, and all the remarkable trainers who tirelessly empower others, transforming lives and uplifting the well-being of countless families.

Your unwavering commitment to mentorship, your passion for helping others succeed, and your selfless dedication to fostering growth and resilience have left an indelible impact on this world. You have not only built thriving teams but also nurtured dreams, inspired hope, and created legacies of empowerment.

Your work goes beyond professional success; it touches the very core of humanity by uplifting those in need and enabling them to achieve their full potential. It is because of leaders like you that the world becomes a better place, one life at a time.

Thank you for your light, your guidance, and your endless belief in the potential of others. This book is a tribute to your extraordinary efforts and the profound difference you continue to make.

With deepest respect and gratitude,
Joseph Gbanabom Conteh

Background of the Book

In a world where financial literacy and strategic planning are the pillars of personal and professional success, *Follow Who Know Road* emerges as a transformative guide for aspiring financial professionals and insurance producers/agents. This book is not just a manual; it is a journey of discovery, empowerment, and mastery of the industry, structured to address six critical questions: **Why? What? How? Who? Where? When?**

Why? Understanding Your WHY

The foundation of success in any endeavor lies in understanding your purpose. *Follow Who Know Road* begins by challenging readers to uncover their "WHY." Why have you chosen to embark on this path? What drives you to pursue a career in financial services or insurance production? By delving into the deeper reasons, such as financial independence, helping others secure their futures, or leaving a legacy, the book helps readers establish a strong emotional and motivational base for their careers.

What? Defining Your Vision, Mission, Goals, and Objectives

Success begins with clarity. This section guides readers to articulate their vision for the future, mission as a professional, and the goals and objectives they seek to achieve. Whether it is becoming a top producer, building a reputable agency, or making a meaningful impact in clients' lives, *Follow Who Know Road* provides tools and strategies to define and align personal and professional aspirations with actionable steps.

How? Achieving Success Through Proven Strategies

Success is not accidental; it is the result of deliberate actions. This section outlines step-by-step strategies for building a thriving financial or insurance business. From networking effectively to mastering product knowledge, understanding market trends, and leveraging technology, readers learn practical skills to excel. The book emphasizes the importance of persistence, adaptability, and continuous learning as cornerstones of professional growth.

Who? Identifying and Following Your Mentor

The title, *Follow Who Know Road,* captures the essence of mentorship. In this section, the book stresses the importance of being coachable and seeking guidance from those who have already succeeded in the field. By attending meetings, asking questions, and actively participating in events, readers are encouraged to surround themselves with mentors and leaders who can provide valuable insights and shortcuts to success.

Where? Accessing Resources for Growth

Every professional journey requires resources—tools, knowledge, and networks. This chapter identifies where readers can access these essentials, such as training programs, industry certifications, books, online resources, and peer communities. It highlights the importance of continuously investing in personal development and staying informed about industry changes to remain competitive.

When? Always Committing to Your Growth

Time is the ultimate resource, and success demands consistent commitment. This final section encourages readers to take control of their time, prioritize their goals, and make continuous progress a daily habit. By setting schedules, maintaining discipline, and embracing a mindset of relentless improvement, Agents can achieve long-term success.

Follow Who Know Road is more than a book—it is a roadmap for anyone seeking growth and fulfillment as a financial professional or insurance agent. By answering the essential questions of *Why, What, How, Who, Where,* and *When,* this book provides readers with the knowledge, strategies, and inspiration to navigate their career paths with confidence and purpose. Whether you are starting out or looking to take your business to new heights, this book is your guide to following the proven road to success.

Table of Contents

Part 1

Meaning, Nature, and scope of Life Insurance Agency Business in the United States and Canada.

Introduction

The life insurance agency business is a vital component of the financial services sector in the United States and Canada, designed to provide individuals and families with financial protection and security. At its core, life insurance offers a safety net, ensuring that beneficiaries receive financial support in the event of the policyholder's death. Agencies and their licensed agents play a crucial role in educating clients about the importance of life insurance, helping them select the right policies tailored to their needs, and fostering long-term relationships to support their evolving financial goals. This business is rooted in trust and responsibility, requiring agents to possess comprehensive product knowledge, strong interpersonal skills, and a deep commitment to serving their clients' best interests.

The scope of the life insurance agency business extends beyond selling policies. Agents often serve as financial advisors, guiding clients in planning for retirement, estate management, wealth transfer, and overall risk mitigation. In the United States and Canada, the industry is highly regulated, ensuring transparency and ethical practices to protect consumers. With advancements in technology, the business has expanded to include digital platforms and tools, making policy selection, underwriting, and claims processing more efficient. Additionally, the growing awareness of financial literacy and the demand for personalized financial solutions have further broadened the opportunities for life insurance agents to make a meaningful impact in their communities while achieving personal and professional growth.

Section I

Meaning of Life Insurance Agency Business in the United States: A Comprehensive Understanding

The **life insurance agency business** in the United States refers to the practice of selling, managing, and servicing life insurance policies. Life insurance itself is a contract between an individual and an insurance company, where the insurer guarantees a sum of money (the death benefit) to the beneficiary upon the insured person's death, in exchange for regular premium payments. The business model of life insurance agencies involves licensed agents acting as intermediaries between clients and insurers, helping individuals and families select the best policies for their financial protection and long-term security. Life insurance agencies play a pivotal role in ensuring that people have access to coverage that can protect loved ones from the financial burdens associated with death, such as loss of income, funeral costs, and outstanding debts.

The **nature** of the life insurance agency business is rooted in service, trust, and risk management. Life insurance agents not only provide advice on selecting appropriate policies but also educate clients about the value of life insurance in the context of overall financial planning, including retirement planning, estate planning, and investment management. Agents are responsible for assessing the needs of clients, presenting suitable policies, and assisting with claims when the need arises. The business operates within a highly regulated environment in the United States, with strict laws and guidelines that govern how life insurance is marketed, sold, and maintained, ensuring consumer protection and ethical practices.

Historical Background

The history of life insurance in the United States dates to the early colonial era. The first life insurance policy in the United States was issued in 1759 by the Presbyterian Ministers Fund in Philadelphia, which was designed to benefit widows and orphans of clergy members. The development of life insurance continued to grow throughout the 19th century as industrialization and urbanization created new financial risks for families. Initially, life insurance policies were reserved for wealthier families, but the growing need for financial security among the working class led to the emergence of a broader market for life insurance.

In the mid-19th century, a series of advancements in actuarial science and the ability to better predict life expectancies and risks helped life insurance become more accessible to the public. The first life insurance company in the U.S., the **Penn Mutual Life Insurance Company**, was founded in 1847, and the industry saw a boom during the late 19th and early 20th centuries, driven by innovations such as the introduction of **industrial life insurance** policies. These policies, which were often sold door-to-door by agents, allowed ordinary people to purchase life insurance in small, affordable increments.

The 20th century marked significant growth in the life insurance industry, particularly after the **Great Depression**. With financial insecurity rampant during the 1930s, many Americans turned to life insurance as a means of protecting their families from potential financial hardships. The establishment of the **Social Security Act of 1935** and subsequent changes in social safety nets further encouraged the need for supplemental life insurance to ensure families' long-term financial security. In the 1940s and 1950s, the rise of employer-sponsored group life insurance further expanded the market for life insurance products.

After World War II, the life insurance business evolved with the development of more diverse products, including **whole life insurance, term**

life insurance, universal life insurance, and **variable life insurance.** The **1960s** also saw the federal government pass significant legislation, such as the **Employee Retirement Income Security Act (ERISA),** which impacted how life insurance policies were integrated into employee benefits plans. The industry continued to expand in the late 20th and early 21st centuries with the growth of **financial planning,** where life insurance became an integral part of broader wealth management strategies.

Today, life insurance agencies are a cornerstone of the U.S. financial services sector. Agents are trained to not only sell life insurance but to act as trusted advisors, offering a wide array of financial solutions to help individuals protect their families, plan for retirement, and ensure their financial legacy. The industry has also adapted to the digital age, with online platforms and technology transforming how agents engage with clients and sell products. The growing awareness of personal finance, estate planning, and the need for long-term financial security has fueled a renewed interest in life insurance, solidifying the role of life insurance agencies as critical players in both the financial landscape and society at large.

In conclusion, the life insurance agency business in the United States has evolved significantly from its early colonial roots. It now encompasses a diverse range of products and services that cater to the varying financial needs of individuals and families. This growth reflects both the increasing awareness of the importance of financial protection and the industry's ongoing efforts to adapt to changing economic, technological, and regulatory environments. Life insurance remains one of the most trusted and essential tools for managing the financial risks associated with death, ensuring that families are safeguarded in their time of need.

Section II

The Nature, and scope of Life Insurance Agency Business in the United States and Canada.

The life insurance agency business in the United States and Canada is a vital part of the financial services sector. This business is primarily focused on providing life insurance coverage to individuals and families, helping them manage the financial risks associated with the death of a policyholder. The business itself involves agents acting as intermediaries between insurance companies and clients, selling life insurance policies, managing customer relations, and advising clients on how to best secure their financial futures. Life insurance agencies work on a commission-based structure, where agents earn commissions based on the policies they sell. In both the U.S. and Canada, life insurance agencies also assist in other financial products such as annuities, disability insurance, and investment solutions, making them integral to personal financial planning.

The nature of the life insurance agency business is rooted in trust, as agents are often tasked with helping clients make decisions about long-term financial security. This includes assessing their financial needs, providing tailored policy options, and ensuring that families are protected from the financial impact of unforeseen events. Agencies in the U.S. and Canada also serve as financial advisors, helping clients plan for retirement, manage estate taxes, and structure wealth transfer strategies. The scope of the business is broad, extending beyond the individual level to include corporate clients and group life insurance policies. Agencies may also offer specialized life insurance products, such as **universal life insurance**, **whole life insurance**, and **term life insurance**, each with different features, benefits, and premium structures.

In both the United States and Canada, life insurance agencies are typically contracted by insurance companies to sell their policies. These agencies operate under various models, including independent agencies, which are not tied to any specific insurer, and exclusive or captive agencies, where agents are restricted to selling products from a single insurer. Independent agents often have the flexibility to offer products from multiple insurance companies, allowing them to provide more diverse options to clients. In contrast, exclusive agencies typically work with one company, but they benefit from the brand recognition and marketing support provided by the insurer. The financial strength of these agencies is often closely tied to the strength of the insurers they represent. Agencies with strong partnerships with financially stable and reputable life insurance companies are better positioned to offer secure, reliable products to their clients.

Several key life insurance companies have shaped the life insurance landscape in the U.S. and Canada, and these companies are renowned for their financial stability and long histories. In the U.S., companies such as **MetLife**, **Prudential Financial**, and **New York Life** are some of the oldest and most prominent players in the life insurance market. **MetLife**, for example, has been in business for over 150 years, having been founded in 1868, and is known for offering a wide range of life insurance products. **Prudential Financial**, established in 1875, is another major insurer that provides comprehensive financial services, including life insurance, retirement planning, and investment solutions. **New York Life**, founded in 1845, is the largest mutual life insurance company in the U.S. and has a strong reputation for its long-term financial strength and customer service. In Canada, **Manulife Financial**, founded in 1887, and **Sun Life Financial**, established in 1865, are two of the leading life insurance companies. Both are well-respected for their comprehensive range of insurance and investment products and have a strong presence in the Canadian market.

The connection between life insurance companies and banks in the U.S. and Canada is significant and has grown stronger over time. Both industries are closely intertwined in the broader financial services sector. Banks often work with life insurance companies to offer complementary products, such as insurance policies and investment products, to their customers. Many banks even distribute life insurance products through their own insurance divisions, allowing them to offer more comprehensive financial services. For example, banks may partner with insurers to provide **credit life insurance** or **mortgage insurance**, which helps cover outstanding loans in the event of the borrower's death. Additionally, some banks acquire life insurance coverage to protect their own financial interests, such as ensuring key employees or mitigating risks associated with their investments. Life insurance can also provide a financial cushion against economic downturns, as it is a stable asset that can be used for long-term investment purposes.

Banks often obtain life insurance coverage to secure their financial health, mitigate risks, and provide benefits to their employees. This coverage can help banks safeguard against the loss of key personnel by providing funds to cover the associated costs. Moreover, life insurance policies, especially **corporate-owned life insurance (COLI)**, are often used by banks to accumulate tax-deferred cash value, which can be used as a financial resource for business expansion or other corporate needs. This use of life insurance is particularly attractive to banks seeking to optimize their balance sheets and secure additional funding sources.

When comparing the financial models of banks and life insurance companies, several distinctions become apparent. Banks primarily generate revenue through interest on loans, deposits, and investment income, while life insurance companies earn income from premiums, underwriting, and investments. Life insurance companies tend to have longer-term financial goals, relying on the accumulation of reserves to pay out death benefits over many years. Banks, on the other hand, often operate on a shorter-term basis, with a focus on liquidity and capital management. Both industries, however, play critical roles in the economy of the U.S. and Canada by facilitating financial security and supporting long-term economic stability. Life insurance companies, through their investments, often provide capital to various sectors of the economy, while banks enable the flow of credit and provide essential financial services to individuals and businesses alike.

In conclusion, the life insurance agency business in the United States and Canada is a key player in the financial sector, offering a range of products that help individuals and families secure their financial futures. With a rich history and a strong connection to both the banking sector and the broader economy, life insurance companies are integral to the financial infrastructure of both countries. Their partnership with banks, as well as their financial strength and stability, ensures that they continue to provide essential services to clients and contribute to the economic well-being of society.

PART 2

The Licensed Life Insurance Agents within the Insurance Industry

Introduction

Licensed life insurance agents are essential professionals within the insurance industry, bridging the gap between complex financial products and the individuals and families who rely on them for security and peace of mind. These agents are not just salespeople; they are trusted advisors who guide clients in making informed decisions to protect their loved ones, build financial resilience, and plan. With expertise in life insurance policies, market trends, and regulatory compliance, licensed agents help clients navigate options ranging from term life to whole life and advanced investment-linked policies. In an ever-evolving industry influenced by economic changes, technological advancements, and shifting consumer needs, licensed life insurance agents remain at the forefront, combining their technical knowledge with empathy and personal service to deliver tailored solutions that meet diverse client goals.

Section III
The Role of Licensed Life Insurance Agents in Financial Planning

Licensed life insurance agents play a crucial role in financial planning, acting as both educators and advisors who help clients navigate complex financial landscapes. Their primary focus extends beyond simply selling policies; they serve as strategic partners, working with individuals, families, and businesses to design comprehensive plans that provide financial security and align with long-term goals.

Assessing Client Needs and Objectives

The process begins with a thorough understanding of the client's unique financial situation. Licensed agents conduct detailed assessments that consider income, expenses, assets, liabilities, and future aspirations. They identify potential financial risks, such as premature death, critical illness, or insufficient savings for retirement. By understanding these factors, agents tailor solutions to bridge gaps and mitigate risks, ensuring clients are well-prepared for life's uncertainties.

Crafting Personalized Solutions

Once the client's needs are identified, licensed agents craft personalized recommendations. For instance, they may suggest term life insurance for young families seeking affordable coverage or whole life insurance for clients interested in policies with cash value accumulation. Agents often integrate these policies into broader financial strategies, ensuring life insurance complements existing investments, retirement plans, and estate planning efforts.

Educating Clients on Financial Products

A critical aspect of an agent's role is demystifying insurance products. Life insurance can be intricate, with varying terms, benefits, and riders. Licensed agents explain these details in plain language, helping clients understand the implications of each option. For example, an agent might highlight the advantages of adding a long-term care rider or discuss how accelerated death benefits can provide financial relief during a terminal illness. By breaking down complex concepts, agents empower clients to make informed decisions.

Supporting Risk Management

Life insurance is a cornerstone of risk management in financial planning. Licensed agents help clients prepare for the unexpected, ensuring their families remain financially secure in the event of a loss. Beyond individual policies, agents also work with business owners to establish key person insurance or buy-sell agreements, safeguarding companies against the financial impact of losing critical personnel.

Facilitating Wealth Transfer and Legacy Planning

Licensed life insurance agents often play a pivotal role in legacy planning, ensuring clients leave behind a financial cushion for their loved ones. They work with estate planners and attorneys to minimize tax liabilities and create strategies for passing wealth efficiently. Life insurance can be an invaluable tool for funding trusts, equalizing inheritances among heirs, or providing liquidity to cover estate taxes and debts.

Staying Updated on Trends and Regulations

The life insurance industry is dynamic, influenced by changes in regulations, market trends, and economic conditions. Licensed agents continually update their knowledge to provide the most relevant advice. For instance, they may recommend policies with inflation-adjusted benefits during times of economic uncertainty or discuss the advantages of newer products like indexed universal life insurance.

Acting as Long-Term Financial Partners

Licensed life insurance agents establish enduring relationships with clients, offering guidance through different life stages. From securing protection for a growing family to optimizing policies in retirement, agents adapt their strategies as clients' circumstances evolve. This long-term approach fosters trust and ensures that financial plans remain aligned with changing goals and needs.

In the intricate world of financial planning, licensed life insurance agents stand out as indispensable allies. Their ability to combine technical expertise with personalized service ensures that clients not only achieve their financial objectives but also gain the peace of mind that comes from being prepared for the future. As the industry continues to evolve, the role of licensed agents will remain vital, helping individuals and families navigate an increasingly complex financial landscape.

Section IV

Trends in Life Insurance Products: What Agents Need to Know

The life insurance industry is undergoing significant transformations, shaped by evolving consumer needs, technological advancements, and regulatory changes. For licensed life insurance agents, staying ahead of these trends is essential to remain competitive and deliver value to their clients. Understanding and adapting to these trends can help agents provide innovative solutions that align with modern financial planning objectives. Here are the key trends that every agent should know:

Rise of Hybrid Life Insurance Products

Hybrid life insurance products, which combine traditional life insurance with additional features like long-term care (LTC) benefits, are gaining popularity. These policies appeal to clients seeking comprehensive coverage in a single product. For instance, a hybrid policy might offer a death benefit while also covering long-term care expenses if the policyholder becomes unable to perform daily living activities. Agents need to understand the nuances of these products to effectively match them with clients who are concerned about rising healthcare costs or who want flexible coverage options.

Growth in Indexed Universal Life (IUL) Policies

Indexed Universal Life policies are becoming increasingly attractive due to their ability to link cash value growth to stock market indices while providing downside protection. Clients looking for a balance between risk and growth potential often find IUL policies appealing. Agents must educate clients on the mechanisms of index credits, caps, and participation rates, while also clarifying that these policies are not direct investments in the stock market.

Increased Demand for Simplified and Accelerated Underwriting

The demand for simplified underwriting processes has grown as consumers seek faster, hassle-free ways to obtain life insurance. Accelerated underwriting, which uses algorithms, big data, and predictive analytics to assess risk without requiring medical exams, is becoming the norm for many insurers. Licensed agents need to familiarize themselves with these technologies and communicate their benefits to clients, particularly those hesitant about traditional underwriting processes.

Focus on Customizable Policies with Add-Ons and Riders

Today's consumers value flexibility and customization. Life insurance policies with a wide range of optional riders—such as critical illness coverage, disability waivers, and return of premium options—are increasingly popular. Agents must understand how these riders work and identify which ones are most suitable for individual clients based on their unique needs and financial goals.

Integration of Technology and Digital Tools

The digital transformation of the insurance industry has introduced tools such as online policy management portals, mobile apps, and wearable technology for health monitoring. Some insurers now offer discounts or incentives for policyholders who use fitness trackers to demonstrate healthy lifestyles. Agents should stay informed about these technological offerings to highlight their benefits to tech-savvy clients.

Growing Interest in Term Life Insurance with Conversion Options

While term life insurance has always been popular due to its affordability, policies with conversion privileges are gaining traction. These allow clients to convert their term policy to permanent life insurance without additional underwriting, offering flexibility as their needs change. Agents can use this feature to address both short-term affordability concerns and long-term planning needs.

Emphasis on Sustainability and Ethical Investments

As more clients prioritize environmental and social responsibility, life insurers are introducing products that align with these values. Policies tied to ethical investments or that contribute to environmental causes (e.g., through carbon offsets) are becoming more common. Licensed agents should be prepared to discuss these options with environmentally conscious clients.

Micro-Insurance and Pay-As-You-Go Policies

In emerging markets and among younger, budget-conscious consumers, micro-insurance and pay-as-you-go policies are on the rise. These products offer affordable coverage with minimal commitment, making life insurance accessible to a broader audience. Agents need to recognize the potential of these offerings to reach underserved or underinsured populations.

Adoption of Blockchain for Transparency and Security

Blockchain technology is beginning to influence the life insurance industry by improving transparency, reducing fraud, and streamlining claims processing. Although still in its early stages, this trend holds significant implications for the agent-client relationship. Agents should stay updated on how blockchain applications can enhance trust and efficiency in policy management.

Life Insurance as a Retirement Tool

With increasing awareness of the retirement savings gap, many clients view life insurance as a dual-purpose tool for protection and supplemental retirement income. Agents must understand how products like permanent life insurance and annuities can provide cash value growth and tax advantages, appealing to clients seeking long-term financial stability.

Post-Pandemic Changes in Consumer Behavior

The COVID-19 pandemic has shifted client priorities, with many placing greater emphasis on financial security and health-related coverage. Agents should adapt their approach to address heightened awareness of mortality risks and the desire for policies that offer accelerated death benefits or critical illness coverage.

Focus on Financial Literacy and Client Education

As clients become more informed and demand transparency, agents are increasingly expected to serve as educators. Providing clear, concise explanations of life insurance options, benefits, and potential drawbacks has become a key aspect of the agent's role. Emphasizing financial literacy can build trust and improve client satisfaction.

For licensed life insurance agents, understanding and adapting to these trends is essential to staying relevant and meeting the evolving needs of their clients. By embracing innovation, leveraging technology, and focusing on client education, agents can continue to play a vital role in securing financial futures and building lasting relationships in an increasingly competitive industry.

Section V

Becoming a Licensed Life Insurance Agent: Steps, Challenges, and Opportunities

Becoming a licensed life insurance agent is a rewarding career path that combines financial expertise, interpersonal skills, and the opportunity to make a meaningful impact on clients' lives. The journey involves several steps to meet licensing requirements, challenges to overcome in building a successful career, and numerous opportunities for professional and personal growth. Here's a comprehensive overview.

Steps to Becoming a Licensed Life Insurance Agent

Understand the Role and Responsibilities

Aspiring agents must first understand the duties of a life insurance agent, which include advising clients, selling policies, and helping people plan for their financial future. Researching the industry and aligning personal goals with the role is a vital first step.

Meet the Basic Requirements

Most states require candidates to be at least 18 years old, have a high school diploma or equivalent, and undergo a background check. Certain states may have additional requirements.

Choose a Life Insurance Focus

Decide whether to specialize in individual life insurance, group policies, or related areas like health insurance or financial planning. This decision will guide the licensing process and career trajectory.

Complete Pre-Licensing Education

Enroll in a state-approved pre-licensing course. These courses cover insurance fundamentals, state regulations, policy types, and ethics. The number of required hours varies by state, typically ranging from 20 to 40 hours.

Pass the Licensing Exam

After completing the coursework, candidates must pass a state-administered life insurance exam. The test assesses knowledge of state regulations, policy structures, and ethical responsibilities. Preparation often involves study guides, practice tests, and review sessions.

Submit an Application and Background Check

Upon passing the exam, candidates must submit a licensing application to their state's insurance department, often accompanied by fingerprints for a background check.

Obtain a State License

Once approved, candidates receive their life insurance license, granting them legal authority to sell policies within the state. Licensing can sometimes extend to other states through reciprocity agreements.

Seek Employment or Start Independently

New agents can join established insurance companies, work as independent agents, or affiliate with brokerage firms. Working for a reputable company often provides training, mentorship, and access to a client base.

Engage in Continuing Education

Most states require licensed agents to complete continuing education (CE) courses periodically to maintain their license and stay updated on industry trends and regulations.

Challenges in Becoming a Licensed Life Insurance Agent

Passing the Licensing Exam

For many, the licensing exam poses a significant hurdle. It requires a strong grasp of technical knowledge and the ability to apply theoretical concepts in practical scenarios.

Building a Client Base

New agents often struggle to establish a network and attract clients. This challenge requires persistence, strategic marketing, and leveraging personal and professional networks.

Adapting to Industry Changes

The insurance industry is constantly evolving due to regulatory updates, technological advancements, and changing consumer expectations. Agents must stay adaptable and proactive in learning.

Handling Rejection

Selling life insurance involves frequent rejections, which can be discouraging for newcomers. Developing resilience and a positive mindset is essential to overcoming this challenge.

Navigating Ethical Dilemmas

Agents must prioritize their clients' best interests while meeting sales targets. Balancing ethical responsibilities with business goals can be a complex aspect of the profession.

Opportunities for Licensed Life Insurance Agents

Career Flexibility and Growth

Life insurance agents have diverse career options, from working with large firms to establishing independent agencies. Success in the field can lead to roles in management, training, or financial advising.

High Earning Potential

Life insurance sales offer competitive commission-based earnings, with significant potential for growth. Experienced agents and those serving high-net-worth clients often enjoy substantial incomes.

Making a Positive Impact

Helping clients secure financial protection for their families is a deeply fulfilling aspect of the job. Agents often develop meaningful relationships with their clients, becoming trusted advisors.

Expanding Knowledge Base

Agents continuously learn about financial planning, investments, estate planning, and tax strategies. This knowledge not only enhances their careers but also enriches their personal financial literacy.

Leveraging Technology

The integration of digital tools like CRM systems, virtual consultations, and predictive analytics enables agents to reach clients more efficiently and provide tailored solutions.

Developing Interpersonal Skills

The role hones communication, negotiation, and relationship-building skills, which are valuable in any professional setting.

Specialization Opportunities

Agents can specialize in areas like business insurance, high-net-worth clients, or group policies, carving a niche that enhances their expertise and marketability.

Becoming a licensed life insurance agent requires dedication, perseverance, and a commitment to professional growth. While the path comes with challenges, it also offers a wealth of opportunities to make a difference in clients' lives and build a rewarding career. By staying informed, embracing innovation, and prioritizing ethical practices, life insurance agents can thrive in an ever-changing industry and achieve both personal and professional success.

Section VI

Ethics and Compliance for Life Insurance Agents

Ethics and compliance are foundational to the life insurance industry, ensuring that agents uphold integrity, build trust with clients, and adhere to legal and regulatory requirements. Life insurance agents operate in a fiduciary capacity, meaning they must prioritize the best interests of their clients while providing transparent and honest guidance. Ethics and compliance not only safeguard the reputation of individual agents and their firms but also protect clients from financial harm and promote public confidence in the insurance sector.

What is Ethics in the Context of Life Insurance?

Ethics in the life insurance industry refers to the moral principles and standards of conduct that guide agents in their professional activities. These principles include honesty, fairness, respect, and accountability. Ethical agents focus on:

Acting in the Client's Best Interest

Recommending policies and solutions that meet the client's needs rather than prioritizing commissions or sales targets.

Transparency in Communication

Providing clear and accurate information about policy terms, conditions, costs, and exclusions to ensure clients make informed decisions.

Maintaining Confidentiality

Protecting sensitive client information and using it only for the purpose of serving their financial and insurance needs.

Avoiding Conflicts of Interest

Disclosing any potential conflicts and ensuring that personal interests do not compromise professional judgment.

What is Compliance in the Context of Life Insurance?

Compliance refers to adherence to the laws, regulations, and industry standards that govern the sale and management of life insurance policies. Regulatory frameworks are designed to protect consumers and ensure fair market practices. For life insurance agents, compliance involves:

Licensing and Continuing Education

Meeting state-specific licensing requirements and completing mandatory continuing education to stay current with industry regulations.

Adherence to Anti-Money Laundering (AML) Laws

Identifying and reporting suspicious financial transactions to prevent the misuse of insurance products for illegal activities.

Following Suitability Standards

Ensuring that recommended policies align with the financial needs, goals, and circumstances of the client.

Compliance with Privacy Laws

Adhering to regulations like the Health Insurance Portability and Accountability Act (HIPAA) and the Gramm-Leach-Bliley Act to safeguard client data.

Avoiding Misrepresentation and Fraud

Refraining from making exaggerated claims or withholding critical information about policies.

Importance of Ethics and Compliance for Life Insurance Agents

Building Client Trust

Ethical practices foster trust and strengthen long-term relationships, which are crucial for client retention and referrals.

Protecting the Agent's Reputation

Compliance with regulations and ethical standards safeguards an agent's professional reputation and reduces the risk of legal consequences.

Promoting Industry Integrity

Ethical behavior and compliance practices enhance public confidence in the insurance industry.

Reducing Legal and Financial Risks

Agents who comply with regulatory requirements are less likely to face penalties, lawsuits, or disciplinary actions.

Enhancing Client Satisfaction

Transparent and honest interactions ensure clients understand their policies, leading to greater satisfaction and fewer disputes.

Common Ethical and Compliance Challenges for Life Insurance Agents

Balancing Sales Goals with Client Interests

Agents may face pressure to meet sales targets, which could tempt them to recommend unsuitable policies.

Complexity of Regulatory Requirements

Staying updated on ever-changing regulations and understanding their implications can be challenging.

Handling Client Misunderstandings

Miscommunication or lack of clarity about policy details can lead to disputes or dissatisfaction.

Pressure from Competitors

Intense competition in the insurance market may drive unethical practices, such as offering misleading information about rival policies.

Strategies to Uphold Ethics and Compliance

Prioritize Client Education

Invest time in helping clients understand their options, including benefits, costs, and limitations of each policy.

Stay Informed

Regularly participate in training, workshops, and continuing education programs to remain current on ethical standards and regulatory requirements.

Use Transparent Sales Practices

Clearly explain commissions, fees, and how policy recommendations align with the client's financial goals.

Implement a Compliance Checklist

Maintain a checklist of key compliance steps, such as completing suitability analyses, obtaining proper client documentation, and adhering to AML requirements.

Seek Guidance When in Doubt

Consult with supervisors, compliance officers, or legal counsel when faced with ethical dilemmas or regulatory ambiguities.

Document All Interactions

Maintain detailed records of client meetings, recommendations, and signed disclosures to provide evidence of ethical conduct.

Ethics and compliance are non-negotiable aspects of a life insurance agent's responsibilities. By adhering to these principles, agents ensure that they provide the highest level of service to clients while protecting themselves and their firms from potential risks. In an industry built on trust and financial security, maintaining ethical integrity and regulatory compliance is not just a professional obligation—it is the foundation of long-term success and a cornerstone of the life insurance profession.

Section VI

Technology and Digital Tools for Life Insurance Agents

The life insurance industry is undergoing a significant digital transformation, reshaping how agents interact with clients, manage their business operations, and deliver personalized services. The adoption of digital platforms, customer relationship management (CRM) tools, and artificial intelligence (AI) has revolutionized the industry, enabling life insurance agents to enhance efficiency, improve client engagement, and provide more tailored solutions. Here's a detailed exploration of these advancements:

1. Digital Platforms for Life Insurance Agents

Digital platforms have streamlined many of the processes involved in selling and managing life insurance policies. These platforms enable agents to connect with clients, process applications, and provide policy updates seamlessly. Key benefits include:

Online Application and Underwriting

Digital platforms simplify the application process by enabling agents to submit forms electronically. Many systems integrate automated underwriting, allowing for quicker approval decisions and reducing the time required to issue policies.

Client Portals

Many insurers now offer portals where clients can view their policies, pay premiums, and update personal information. Agents can use these portals to keep clients engaged and informed, reducing administrative burdens.

E-Signatures and Document Management

The adoption of e-signature technology allows clients to sign policy documents electronically, speeding up transactions and enhancing convenience. Digital document management systems help agents store and retrieve policy information efficiently.

Mobile Apps

Mobile apps provide agents with on-the-go access to policy details, customer interactions, and performance analytics, ensuring they remain productive and responsive, even in the field.

2. Customer Relationship Management (CRM) Tools

CRM tools are indispensable for modern life insurance agents, offering a centralized system to manage client relationships and track interactions. These tools have transformed the way agents engage with clients, providing insights and automation that drive efficiency and personalization.

Client Data Management
CRM tools store detailed client profiles, including personal information, communication history, and policy details. This allows agents to provide more personalized recommendations and maintain a consistent relationship with clients.

Automated Reminders and Follow-Ups
CRM tools can schedule automatic reminders for premium payments, policy renewals, or annual reviews, ensuring that agents never miss an opportunity to connect with clients.

Sales Funnel Tracking
Agents can use CRM systems to monitor the progress of leads through the sales pipeline, helping them identify high-priority prospects and optimize their sales efforts.

Analytics and Reporting
Advanced CRM tools offer analytics that provide insights into client behaviors, policy trends, and agent performance. This data helps agents refine their strategies and identify new opportunities for growth.

3. Artificial Intelligence (AI) in Life Insurance

AI is revolutionizing the life insurance industry by enhancing efficiency, accuracy, and client experience. For agents, AI-powered tools provide significant advantages in various aspects of their work.

Predictive Analytics

AI can analyze historical data to predict client needs and preferences. For example, it might identify clients likely to be interested in policy upgrades or additional coverage, enabling agents to tailor their outreach.

Chatbots and Virtual Assistants

AI-driven chatbots can handle routine client inquiries, such as policy details or premium payment schedules, freeing up agents to focus on more complex tasks. Virtual assistants can also help agents manage their schedules, send reminders, and provide quick access to policy information.

Automated Underwriting

AI-powered underwriting systems assess risks more accurately by analyzing vast amounts of data, including medical records and financial histories. This not only speeds up the underwriting process but also ensures fair and consistent decision-making.

Personalized Recommendations

AI algorithms can evaluate a client's financial situation, risk tolerance, and life stage to suggest the most suitable policies. This enhances the client experience and improves the likelihood of policy acceptance.

Fraud Detection

AI tools are adept at detecting fraudulent activities by analyzing patterns and anomalies in policy applications and claims. This protects agents and insurers from financial losses and ensures compliance with regulatory standards.

4. Benefits of Technology and Digital Tools for Agents

The integration of technology into the life insurance industry has brought numerous benefits for agents:

Improved Efficiency

Automation reduces the time spent on administrative tasks, allowing agents to focus on client interactions and business development.

Enhanced Client Engagement

Digital tools enable agents to communicate with clients more frequently and effectively, fostering stronger relationships.

Increased Accuracy

AI and digital platforms minimize human errors

in data entry, underwriting, and claims processing, ensuring smoother transactions.

Greater Reach

Online marketing tools and virtual meeting platforms allow agents to connect with clients beyond geographical boundaries, expanding their potential client base.

Adaptability to Changing Consumer Expectations

Today's clients demand convenience, speed, and transparency. Digital tools enable agents to meet these expectations by offering streamlined and accessible services.

5. Challenges and Considerations

While technology offers immense benefits, it also poses challenges that agents must address:

Learning Curve

Agents must invest time and effort to learn and adapt to new tools and technologies.

Data Security

With increased reliance on digital tools, protecting sensitive client information from cyber threats becomes paramount.

Balancing Technology with Personal Touch

While automation enhances efficiency, agents

must ensure that their interactions remain personalized and empathetic.

6. Future of Technology in Life Insurance

The role of technology in the life insurance industry will continue to grow, with emerging trends such as:

Blockchain for Policy Management
Blockchain technology can improve transparency, security, and efficiency in managing policies and claims.

Internet of Things (IoT) Integration
IoT devices, such as wearable fitness trackers, can provide real-time data on client health, enabling personalized policy pricing and risk assessment.

Voice and Biometric Technologies
Voice recognition and biometric tools may simplify client authentication and policy access.

Enhanced AI Capabilities
Advanced AI algorithms will offer even more precise insights and automation, further improving client service and business outcomes.

Technology and digital tools have fundamentally transformed the way life insurance agents operate, empowering them to serve clients with greater efficiency, accuracy, and personalization. By embracing these advancements, agents can stay competitive in a rapidly evolving industry, build stronger client relationships, and achieve sustainable growth. However, to fully leverage these tools, agents must stay informed, invest in continuous learning, and strike a balance between technological efficiency and the human touch that remains central to their profession.

Section VII

Marketing Strategies for Licensed Life Insurance Agents

Marketing is a vital aspect of success for licensed life insurance agents, as it helps attract clients, build trust, and establish a competitive edge in the industry. Effective strategies involve building a personal brand, leveraging social media, and creating client-focused campaigns to meet the evolving needs of clients and the market.

Building a personal brand starts with defining a niche. Agents must identify the specific audience or market segment they want to serve, such as young families, retirees, or business owners. Specializing in areas like estate planning or retirement solutions helps differentiate them from competitors. A unique value proposition (UVP) is also crucial, as it highlights what sets the agent apart, such as their expertise in simplifying complex policies or providing a compassionate approach. A consistent brand image is essential across all materials, including business cards, social media profiles, and websites. Testimonials and success stories showcasing positive client experiences add credibility to the brand. Agents who consistently educate their audience through resources like eBooks, newsletters, or webinars further enhance their reputation as experts in the field.

Social media platforms are powerful tools for connecting with clients and building professional credibility. LinkedIn is ideal for thought leadership, as agents can share articles, post industry updates, and network with professionals. On Facebook, creating a professional business page for testimonials and updates and using targeted ads helps reach specific demographics. Instagram allows agents to share visually appealing content like infographics and engage clients with interactive stories and reels. YouTube provides a platform for educational videos, such as tutorials and answers to frequently asked questions. Twitter can be used for quick tips and participating in trending discussions. Consistency is key when using social media. Agents must post regularly, use relevant hashtags, and respond to comments and messages promptly. Analytics tools on these platforms enable agents to track engagement and refine their strategies for better results.

Creating client-focused campaigns is another critical aspect of successful marketing. These campaigns prioritize the needs and concerns of the target audience. Personalized messaging is essential, as it demonstrates that agents understand their clients' unique goals.

Educational content, such as articles and videos answering common questions about life insurance, builds trust and positions the agent as a knowledgeable resource. Storytelling is a powerful technique for connecting with clients emotionally, as sharing real-life examples of how life insurance has impacted others can resonate deeply. Seasonal and event-based campaigns, such as promoting financial planning during tax season or retirement readiness month, help align marketing efforts with timely themes. Clear calls-to-action (CTAs) like Schedule a free consultation or attend our webinar guide potential clients toward the next step.

In addition to these core strategies, agents can enhance their marketing efforts through networking and community engagement. Attending local events, sponsoring activities, and partnering with other professionals such as financial advisors or real estate agents can increase visibility and generate referrals. Online reviews and client referrals are also valuable, as satisfied clients can recommend the agent to their networks. Search engine optimization (SEO) ensures the agent's website ranks higher on search engines, making it easier for potential clients to find them. Paid advertising on platforms like Google and Facebook can target specific audiences, while retargeting campaigns help engage individuals who have previously shown interest.

Licensed life insurance agents must prioritize trust, value, and engagement in their marketing strategies. By focusing on personal branding, leveraging the power of social media, and designing client-focused campaigns, agents can effectively connect with their audience and establish themselves as reliable professionals. Incorporating digital tools and innovative approaches ensures agents remain competitive and thrive in a rapidly changing industry.

Section VIII

Navigating Complex Cases: High-Net-Worth Clients and Advanced Life Insurance Needs

Serving high-net-worth clients with advanced life insurance needs requires a sophisticated approach that combines technical expertise, personalized service, and a deep understanding of complex financial strategies. These clients often have multifaceted financial profiles, diverse investment portfolios, and unique goals, such as wealth preservation, estate planning, and tax mitigation. Life insurance agents catering to this market must be adept at navigating these complexities while delivering tailored solutions that align with their clients' overarching financial objectives.

High-net-worth individuals (HNWIs) typically use life insurance as a versatile tool to address a range of financial needs. Unlike traditional clients who may view life insurance primarily to provide for dependents, HNWIs often see it as an integral component of their wealth management strategies. For these clients, life insurance can serve as a vehicle for wealth transfer, liquidity creation, business succession planning, and charitable giving. Agents must, therefore, approach these cases with a broader perspective, integrating insurance solutions into the client's overall financial ecosystem.

Estate planning is one of the most critical areas where life insurance plays a pivotal role for high-net-worth clients. Given the potential for substantial estate taxes, especially in jurisdictions with high thresholds, HNWIs often rely on life insurance policies to provide liquidity for their heirs to settle tax obligations without selling off valuable assets. Life insurance trusts, such as irrevocable life insurance trusts (ILITs), are commonly used to hold policies outside the taxable estate, ensuring that the death benefit is not subject to estate taxes. Agents working in this space must collaborate with estate attorneys and financial advisors to structure these trusts effectively and comply with regulatory requirements.

Tax efficiency is another primary concern for high-net-worth clients, and life insurance offers unique advantages in this regard. Permanent life insurance policies, such as whole life or indexed universal life (IUL), provide tax-deferred cash value growth, which can be accessed through loans or withdrawals. These policies can serve as a supplemental retirement income source, enabling clients to minimize taxable distributions from other accounts. Advanced strategies, such as premium financing, may also appeal to

HNWIs, allowing them to leverage their assets to fund large life insurance premiums while preserving liquidity. Agents must have a thorough understanding of these strategies, including their risks and benefits, to guide clients appropriately.

For business owners, life insurance is often a cornerstone of business succession planning. HNWIs who own businesses may require policies to fund buy-sell agreements, ensuring a smooth transition of ownership in the event of a partner's death. Key person insurance is another critical tool, providing financial stability to the business if a key executive or owner passes away. Agents must understand the intricacies of these policies and work closely with business advisors to ensure that the insurance solutions align with the overall succession plan.

Charitable giving is another area where high-net-worth clients leverage life insurance. By naming a charity as the beneficiary of a life insurance policy, clients can create a lasting philanthropic legacy while also enjoying potential tax benefits. Alternatively, clients may donate the policy itself or use the death benefit to fund charitable trusts. Navigating these arrangements requires agents to be well-versed in the legal and financial implications of charitable planning to provide informed advice.

One of the challenges of working with high-net-worth clients is the need for customization and precision. These clients expect tailored solutions that address their unique circumstances. Agents must conduct comprehensive assessments of their clients' financial situations, goals, and risk tolerance levels. This often involves gathering detailed information about their assets, liabilities, income streams, and family dynamics. A collaborative approach is essential, as agents frequently work alongside accountants, attorneys, and wealth managers to ensure a cohesive strategy.

Communication is another critical factor when serving high-net-worth clients. These individuals are often highly informed and accustomed to working with financial professionals, so agents must be able to articulate complex insurance solutions clearly and confidently. Regular reviews and updates are also necessary, as the financial needs and priorities of HNWIs can evolve over time due to changes in tax laws, economic conditions, or personal circumstances. Providing proactive and ongoing service helps build trust and reinforces the agent's value.

Technology also plays a significant role in managing complex cases. Advanced customer relationship management (CRM) systems allow agents to track client interactions, document preferences, and monitor policy performance effectively. Data analytics tools can help identify opportunities for policy optimization or suggest additional coverage options based on the client's financial profile. Agents must embrace these technologies to deliver a high level of service and stay ahead in a competitive market.

In conclusion, serving high-net-worth clients with advanced life insurance needs requires a combination of technical expertise, strategic thinking, and personalized attention. Agents must navigate complex financial scenarios, collaborate with other professionals, and remain adaptable to the dynamic nature of their clients' needs. By mastering the intricacies of estate planning, tax efficiency, business succession, and charitable giving, agents can position themselves as trusted advisors who provide invaluable support to their high-net-worth clients. This not only enhances client satisfaction but also solidifies the agent's reputation as a specialist in addressing the unique challenges of this demanding market segment.

Section IX

Continuing Education and Professional Development for Life Insurance Agents

Continuing education (CE) and professional development are critical for life insurance agents who aim to remain competitive, compliant, and effective in a constantly evolving industry. The insurance landscape is shaped by changing regulations, emerging technologies, innovative product offerings, and shifts in consumer expectations. To succeed, agents must embrace lifelong learning and invest in their professional growth to stay informed, build expertise, and provide superior service to clients.

Regulatory compliance is one of the primary drivers of continuing education for life insurance agents. Most states mandate that licensed agents complete periodic continuing education courses to renew their licenses. These requirements ensure that agents remain knowledgeable about state-specific laws, industry standards, and ethical guidelines. Topics often include updates on tax laws affecting life insurance, anti-money laundering (AML) regulations, and consumer protection practices. By fulfilling these CE requirements, agents not only maintain their licensure but also demonstrate a commitment to ethical and legal compliance, which is crucial for building trust with clients.

Beyond regulatory requirements, professional development allows agents to deepen their expertise and expand their skill sets. Advanced certifications and designations, such as the Chartered Life Underwriter (CLU), Certified Financial Planner (CFP), and Life Underwriter Training Council Fellow (LUTCF), provide agents with specialized knowledge in areas like estate planning, retirement solutions, and financial advising. These credentials not only enhance an agent's credibility but also open doors to serving high-net-worth clients or addressing complex financial needs. By pursuing such qualifications, agents position themselves as trusted advisors who can offer holistic solutions rather than merely selling insurance products.

In addition to formal certifications, agents benefit from attending workshops, seminars, and industry conferences. These events provide opportunities to learn from experts, gain insights into emerging trends, and network with peers. Conferences often cover topics such as technological innovations in the insurance sector, new product developments, and strategies for improving client engagement. Exposure to diverse perspectives and case studies can inspire agents to adopt innovative practices in their own businesses.

The rapid pace of technological advancement in the insurance industry underscores the importance of ongoing education. Digital tools, such as customer relationship management (CRM) software, data analytics, and artificial intelligence (AI), are transforming how agents operate and serve clients. Continuing education programs that focus on technology integration can help agents streamline their workflows, enhance client interactions, and leverage data to make informed decisions. For example, learning to use predictive analytics tools allows agents to identify client needs proactively, while mastering digital marketing platforms helps agents expand their reach and attract new clients.

Staying updated on product knowledge is another critical aspect of professional development. The life insurance market is dynamic, with insurers regularly introducing new policy options, riders, and benefits. Agents must understand these innovations to recommend the most suitable solutions to their clients. For instance, products like indexed universal life (IUL) insurance or hybrid policies that combine life insurance with long-term care benefits require agents to understand their structure, risks, and advantages thoroughly. By keeping up with these developments, agents can differentiate themselves in a competitive market and offer tailored recommendations that meet clients' evolving needs.

Soft skills development is equally important for life insurance agents. While technical knowledge is essential, the ability to communicate effectively, build rapport, and empathize with clients is what truly sets successful agents apart. Continuing education programs often include training in active listening, negotiation, and presentation skills, all of which are critical for understanding client concerns and building trust. Additionally, courses on emotional intelligence and cultural competence enable agents to connect with diverse client populations, fostering inclusive and personalized service.

Professional development also includes cultivating leadership and business management skills. For agents who aspire to grow their practices or lead teams, learning about strategic planning, marketing, and operations management is invaluable. Business-focused courses can teach agents how to optimize their workflows, manage client portfolios effectively, and scale their businesses. Leadership training helps agents mentor junior colleagues, foster collaboration, and inspire their teams to achieve shared goals.

Another vital aspect of continuing education is client education and engagement. As clients become more informed and tech-savvy, they expect transparency and clarity when discussing financial products. Agents who invest in professional development programs that emphasize educational techniques can better explain complex policies, address misconceptions, and empower clients to make informed decisions. This not only enhances client satisfaction but also strengthens long-term relationships.

Networking is a key component of professional growth, and continuing education often facilitates valuable connections. Whether through online forums, in-person workshops, or industry associations, agents can share experiences, exchange ideas, and collaborate on solutions to common challenges. Building a robust professional network also creates opportunities for mentorship, partnerships, and referrals, all of which contribute to career advancement.

In conclusion, continuing education and professional development are indispensable for life insurance agents seeking to excel in a competitive and rapidly evolving industry. By staying compliant with regulatory requirements, pursuing advanced certifications, mastering new technologies, and refining their soft skills, agents can enhance their expertise and provide exceptional service to their clients. Investing in professional growth not only ensures career longevity but also solidifies an agent's reputation as a knowledgeable, trustworthy, and forward-thinking professional. This commitment to lifelong learning ultimately benefits clients, strengthens the agent-client relationship, and contributes to the overall integrity of the life insurance industry.

Section X

The Impact of Economic Shifts on Life Insurance Sales

What Economic Factors Like Inflation, Interest Rates, and Employment Trends Influence Demand

Economic shifts significantly impact life insurance sales, shaping consumer behavior, influencing policy design, and altering industry dynamics. Life insurance, being both a protection tool and a financial product, is closely tied to broader economic conditions. Factors such as inflation, interest rates, and employment trends directly affect the demand for life insurance, as well as the strategies agents and insurers use to adapt to changing economic realities. Understanding these influences is critical for agents to navigate fluctuations in demand and offer relevant solutions to clients.

Inflation and Its Impact on Life Insurance Sales

Inflation, which erodes the purchasing power of money over time, plays a significant role in the life insurance market. During periods of high inflation, consumers may prioritize immediate financial needs over long-term planning, leading to reduced demand for life insurance. Rising costs of living make it harder for individuals to allocate discretionary income to premiums, especially for middle- and lower-income households.

For those who maintain life insurance coverage, inflation can diminish the real value of the death benefit, as the fixed payout may no longer be sufficient to cover future financial needs. This concern increases demand for policies with inflation-protection features, such as indexed universal life insurance (IUL), which ties cash value growth to inflation-adjusted indices.

Agents must address these concerns by educating clients about inflation's impact and recommending policies that include riders or benefits designed to preserve value in inflationary environments. Additionally, they may suggest hybrid products or investment-linked policies that offer potential growth tied to inflation-resistant assets.

Interest Rates and Their Role in Life Insurance Sales

Interest rates have a profound effect on the life insurance industry, influencing both consumer behavior and the profitability of insurers. When interest rates rise, insurers earn higher returns on their investments, often leading to more competitive pricing and attractive policy features. Policies with cash value components, such as whole life and universal life insurance, become more appealing because they offer higher credited interest rates.

Conversely, in low-interest-rate environments, insurers face reduced investment returns, which may lead to higher premiums or lower guarantees on policies. For consumers, this can reduce the perceived value of certain products, particularly those with a strong savings or investment component.

Interest rates also affect consumer decision-making. During high-interest-rate periods, consumers may opt for alternative investment products that offer higher returns than life insurance policies with cash value. On the other hand, in low-rate environments, life insurance policies with guaranteed returns can appear more attractive as a secure savings vehicle.

Agents must stay informed about interest rate trends and adjust their recommendations accordingly. They should focus on highlighting the benefits of guaranteed coverage during periods of low rates and emphasize growth potential in high-rate environments.

Employment Trends and Their Influence on Life Insurance Demand

Employment trends significantly impact life insurance sales, as income stability and access to employer-sponsored benefits are closely linked to consumers' ability to purchase and maintain coverage. High levels of employment and rising wages generally lead to increased demand for life insurance, as individuals are more confident in their financial stability and more likely to plan for long-term needs. Employer-sponsored group life insurance policies often serve as an entry point for many individuals into the life insurance market, creating opportunities for agents to upsell or cross-sell additional coverage.

In contrast, periods of high unemployment or economic downturns can suppress life insurance sales. Job losses often result in lapses in coverage for individuals who depend on employer-sponsored plans, and economic uncertainty may discourage discretionary spending on individual policies. For those who remain employed, concerns about job security may prompt interest in term life insurance, which offers coverage at a lower cost compared to permanent policies.

Agents should adapt their strategies during economic downturns by focusing on affordable options, such as term policies or simplified issue life insurance. These products can provide essential coverage without significant financial strain, helping clients maintain financial protection during uncertain times.

Broader Economic Factors Affecting Life Insurance Sales

Several broader economic trends also play a role in shaping the life insurance market. For example, consumer confidence directly influences purchasing decisions. When confidence in the economy is high, individuals are more likely to invest in long-term financial products like life insurance. Conversely, during periods of economic uncertainty, consumers may delay purchasing decisions or opt for minimal coverage.

Additionally, demographic, and societal shifts, such as aging populations or changes in family structures, interact with economic trends to influence life insurance demand. For instance, younger generations may delay purchasing life insurance due to rising student debt or delayed homeownership, trends often exacerbated by broader economic conditions. Agents must account for these demographic nuances and address the specific financial concerns of different client segments.

Strategies for Agents to Navigate Economic Shifts

Adapting to economic shifts requires life insurance agents to remain flexible, informed, and proactive in addressing client needs. During inflationary periods, agents should focus on educating clients about the erosion of purchasing power and recommend policies with inflation-resistant features. In low-interest-rate environments, they can highlight the benefits of guaranteed protection and explore hybrid or investment-linked products that offer growth potential.

When unemployment rises or economic uncertainty looms, agents should prioritize affordability and accessibility. Simplified issue policies, term life insurance, or policies with flexible premium options can appeal to clients facing financial constraints. Additionally, agents should emphasize the importance of maintaining at least basic coverage to avoid gaps that could jeopardize long-term financial security.

Agents also benefit from staying updated on economic trends through continuing education and leveraging technology to analyze market data. This knowledge allows them to anticipate client concerns and proactively offer solutions. Building strong relationships with clients during challenging economic times can foster trust and loyalty, positioning the agent as a reliable advisor regardless of external conditions.

Economic shifts, including inflation, interest rate changes, and employment trends, profoundly influence life insurance sales and client behavior. Understanding these factors enables agents to adapt their strategies and provide relevant, value-driven solutions that address clients' evolving financial needs. By staying informed, flexible, and client-focused, life insurance agents can successfully navigate the challenges and opportunities presented by economic changes, ensuring both their clients' financial security and their own professional success.

Section XI

Life Insurance and Retirement Planning: An Agent's Perspective

Life Insurance and Retirement Planning: An Agent's Perspective

Life insurance plays a critical role in retirement planning, offering a unique combination of financial security, income supplementation, and wealth transfer benefits. From an agent's perspective, the challenge lies in helping clients understand how life insurance extends beyond traditional risk protection to become a valuable component of their retirement strategy. By integrating life insurance into a comprehensive financial plan, agents can address clients' long-term goals while providing solutions that align with their risk tolerance, income needs, and legacy objectives.

One of the most significant ways life insurance supports retirement planning is through its potential to supplement income. Permanent life insurance policies, such as whole life or universal life, accumulate cash value over time. This cash value grows on a tax-deferred basis and can be accessed during retirement to provide an additional income stream. Agents help clients strategically structure these policies to ensure sufficient cash value growth while protecting the death benefit. This approach is particularly valuable for individuals concerned about outliving their retirement savings or facing unexpected expenses in later years.

Agents also educate clients on the tax advantages of life insurance as a retirement planning tool. Withdrawals or loans taken against the cash value of a policy are typically tax-free, provided the policy is structured correctly and the guidelines are followed. This feature allows clients to access funds without triggering additional tax liabilities, unlike distributions from traditional retirement accounts such as 401(k)s or IRAs. For high-net-worth individuals, these tax benefits make life insurance an attractive option for diversifying their retirement income sources and reducing overall tax exposure.

In addition to providing income, life insurance can serve as a safeguard for retirement assets. Agents often emphasize the importance of protecting a client's retirement savings against unforeseen circumstances, such as medical emergencies, long-term care needs, or market volatility. Certain policies offer riders that allow clients to access the death benefit early to cover critical illness or long-term care expenses. These features ensure that clients can manage unexpected costs without depleting their primary retirement accounts, preserving their financial stability throughout retirement.

Agents also help clients use life insurance as part of their legacy planning. For many, retirement is not only about sustaining their lifestyle but also about leaving a financial legacy for loved ones. Life insurance provides a guaranteed death benefit that can be passed on to heirs, ensuring that the client's wealth is preserved and transferred efficiently. This benefit is particularly valuable for individuals who wish to protect their estate from taxes or equalize inheritances among beneficiaries. For example, an agent might recommend a life insurance policy to provide liquidity for estate taxes, allowing other assets, such as property or investments, to remain intact for heirs.

Moreover, agents play a crucial role in customizing life insurance solutions to fit the unique needs of retirees. For clients nearing or already in retirement, the focus often shifts from wealth accumulation to asset preservation and income stability. Agents help clients evaluate their options, such as converting term life insurance to permanent policies, optimizing existing coverage, or adding features like guaranteed income riders. These adjustments ensure that the policies remain relevant and aligned with the client's evolving priorities.

Another key area where agents provide value is in addressing the longevity risk many retirees face. With life expectancy increasing, clients are often concerned about whether their retirement savings will last throughout their lifetime. Life insurance can act as a financial bridge, providing funds to supplement income or cover unexpected expenses during the later stages of retirement. Agents highlight how life insurance offers peace of mind by addressing this uncertainty, enabling clients to enjoy their retirement without constantly worrying about depleting their resources.

From an agent's perspective, building trust and fostering education are essential when discussing life insurance and retirement planning. Clients often have misconceptions about life insurance, viewing it solely as a tool for income replacement during their working years. Agents must take the time to explain the broader benefits of life insurance, demonstrating how it complements other retirement strategies, such as investments and annuities. Clear communication, personalized recommendations, and a focus on long-term value are crucial for helping clients see the bigger picture.

Agents also collaborate with other financial professionals, such as financial planners and estate attorneys, to create holistic plans that integrate life insurance with the client's overall retirement strategy. This team-based approach ensures that all aspects of the client's financial well-being are addressed, from tax planning to asset allocation. By working closely with other experts, agents can provide more comprehensive and tailored solutions.

In conclusion, life insurance is a versatile and indispensable tool in retirement planning, offering income supplementation, tax advantages, asset protection, and legacy benefits. From an agent's perspective, the role involves educating clients, customizing solutions, and integrating life insurance into a broader financial strategy. By demonstrating the value of life insurance in achieving financial security and addressing retirement goals, agents empower clients to navigate retirement with confidence and peace of mind. This approach not only ensures the client's financial well-being but also reinforces the agent's position as a trusted advisor in the client's financial journey.

Section XII

Strategies for Agents to Overcome Client Objections to Life Insurance

Overcoming client objections to life insurance requires a combination of empathy, education, and effective communication. Many clients hesitate to purchase life insurance due to misconceptions, financial concerns, or a lack of understanding about its importance. For life insurance agents, addressing these objections means not only presenting facts but also connecting emotionally with clients and tailoring solutions to their unique needs. By employing proven prospecting techniques and refining their communication skills, agents can guide hesitant clients toward making informed and confident decisions about life insurance.

The first step in overcoming objections is understanding the underlying reasons for a client's hesitation. Clients may object to life insurance due to cost concerns, perceived complexity, or an underestimation of their own financial risks. For example, some clients may feel that life insurance premiums are an unnecessary expense, while others may believe they don't need coverage because they are young, healthy, or single. Agents must listen attentively to identify these concerns, showing empathy and patience while refraining from making assumptions about the client's objections.

A key technique for addressing objections is education. Many clients simply lack the information they need to make an informed decision. Agents should focus on explaining the benefits of life insurance in clear, relatable terms, emphasizing how it provides financial security for loved ones, covers final expenses, or serves as a tool for wealth building. For instance, agents can illustrate scenarios where life insurance ensures a family's financial stability after an unexpected loss or helps pay off debts like mortgages and student loans. These examples create a tangible understanding of the product's value and help clients see life insurance as a proactive, protective measure rather than a cost.

Personalization is another powerful strategy. Generic pitches are unlikely to resonate with clients who view life insurance as irrelevant to their circumstances. Agents should tailor their approach by using client-specific examples and showing how life insurance aligns with the client's financial goals. For instance, a young professional might be interested in term life insurance to protect their family from future debt, while a retiree might value a permanent policy as part of an estate planning strategy. Personalized recommendations demonstrate that the agent has taken the time to understand the client's situation, fostering trust and increasing the likelihood of overcoming objections.

Storytelling is an effective way to connect emotionally with clients and address their objections. Sharing real-life examples of how life insurance has helped other individuals or families can make the benefits more relatable and compelling. For instance, an agent might describe a situation where a family avoided financial hardship because of life insurance or highlight how a policy enabled a business owner to secure their company's future. These stories create an emotional connection that helps clients see the importance of life insurance in their own lives.

Proactively addressing potential objections before they arise is another useful technique. Agents can anticipate common concerns, such as affordability, and provide solutions upfront. For example, an agent might explain how term life insurance offers affordable coverage with the option to convert to a permanent policy later. By addressing these issues preemptively, agents can reduce resistance and position themselves as knowledgeable and proactive advisors.

Effective questioning techniques are essential for uncovering the client's underlying needs and addressing objections. Open-ended questions encourage clients to share their concerns and priorities, enabling agents to respond with tailored solutions. For instance, an agent might ask, "What financial goals are most important to you?" or "How would you like to ensure your family is taken care of in the future?" These questions shift the focus to the client's objectives, making it easier to demonstrate how life insurance fits into their overall financial plan.

Providing clear, straightforward comparisons of policy options can help clients overcome objections related to complexity. Many clients find the variety of life insurance products overwhelming, which can lead to indecision or resistance. Agents should break down the differences between term and permanent insurance, explaining their respective advantages and disadvantages in simple terms. Visual aids, such as charts or infographics, can further clarify the options and make the decision-making process less intimidating.

Building trust is critical for overcoming objections. Clients are more likely to consider life insurance if they believe the agent genuinely has their best interests at heart. Agents should prioritize transparency, openly discussing the costs, benefits, and limitations of different policies. They should also emphasize their role as a trusted advisor, committed to helping clients achieve long-term financial security. Following up with clients and maintaining consistent communication reinforces this trust, even if the client does not immediately commit to a policy.

Handling affordability objections requires creative solutions. When clients express concern about the cost of life insurance, agents can focus on the flexibility of coverage options. For example, they might recommend starting with a smaller term policy and gradually increasing coverage as the client's financial situation improves. Explaining the cost of inaction—such as the financial burden on loved ones in the absence of coverage—can also help clients understand the value of life insurance relative to its cost.

Agents should also address misconceptions about life insurance that fuel objections. For instance, some clients may believe they are too young or healthy to need coverage, while others may think life insurance is only necessary for those with dependents. Agents can dispel these myths by highlighting the advantages of locking in lower premiums while young and the broader uses of life insurance, such as covering final expenses or serving as a financial asset.

Finally, agents must adopt a long-term perspective. Overcoming objections is not always about closing a sale during the first meeting. Building relationships, providing ongoing education, and demonstrating genuine care for the client's well-being can eventually turn hesitancy into trust. By staying patient and consistent, agents increase the likelihood of converting prospects into lifelong clients.

In summary, overcoming objections to life insurance requires a multifaceted approach that combines empathy, education, and strategic communication. By understanding client concerns, personalizing recommendations, and proactively addressing potential objections, agents can guide hesitant clients toward recognizing the value of life insurance. Techniques such as storytelling, open-ended questioning, and trust-building reinforce the agent's role as a trusted advisor, ultimately helping clients make informed decisions that secure their financial futures.

Section XIII

Diversity and Inclusion in the Life Insurance Agent Workforce

Exploring Efforts to Attract and Retain Diverse Talent in the Life Insurance Sector

Diversity and inclusion are becoming central to the growth and success of the life insurance industry. As societies become more diverse, the need for a workforce that reflects this diversity is essential for meeting the unique needs of a wide range of clients. Attracting and retaining diverse talent in the life insurance sector involves addressing systemic challenges, creating equitable opportunities, and fostering an inclusive culture where agents from all backgrounds can thrive. Efforts to promote diversity and inclusion not only benefit employees but also enhance the industry's ability to connect with underrepresented markets and provide tailored financial solutions.

One of the driving forces behind the push for diversity in the life insurance workforce is the evolving demographic landscape. Populations are increasingly multicultural, with significant growth in minority and immigrant communities. These groups often have unique financial goals, cultural values, and perspectives on life insurance. A diverse agent workforce is better equipped to understand and address these needs, as agents who share cultural or linguistic similarities with clients can build trust and create personalized solutions more effectively.

Attracting diverse talent to the life insurance industry requires intentional strategies. Many life insurance companies have recognized the importance of broadening their recruitment efforts to reach candidates from underrepresented groups. Partnerships with historically Black colleges and universities (HBCUs), Hispanic-serving institutions, and organizations that support women and LGBTQ+ professionals are examples of targeted recruitment initiatives. These partnerships help life insurance companies identify and engage talented individuals who may not have previously considered careers in the industry.

In addition to outreach, companies are focusing on creating accessible pathways into the profession. Internship programs, scholarships, and mentorship opportunities for individuals from underrepresented backgrounds provide valuable exposure to the industry and reduce barriers to entry. For example, mentoring programs pair experienced agents with newcomers, offering guidance, skill development, and career advancement opportunities. Such initiatives not only attract talent but also demonstrate a commitment to fostering long-term success for individuals from diverse communities.

Retention of diverse talent is equally critical and often requires companies to address workplace culture and systemic barriers. Inclusive workplaces are those where all employees feel valued, respected, and supported. To achieve this, life insurance companies are investing in diversity and inclusion training to raise awareness of unconscious bias, promote cultural competency, and foster a sense of belonging among employees. Leadership development programs aimed at underrepresented groups also help ensure that diverse agents have opportunities to advance into leadership positions, further strengthening the industry's commitment to inclusion.

Creating a supportive environment for diverse agents includes offering flexibility and resources that address unique challenges. For example, agents with caregiving responsibilities may benefit from flexible work arrangements, while those from historically marginalized communities may require additional mentorship or networking opportunities to navigate the industry successfully. Companies that prioritize mental health and well-being initiatives also contribute to a workplace culture where diverse agents feel empowered to succeed.

In addition to internal efforts, life insurance companies are working to expand their outreach to underserved communities. Agents from diverse backgrounds often play a vital role in bridging the gap between these communities and the industry. By understanding cultural norms and financial priorities specific to their communities, diverse agents can create marketing campaigns, educational workshops, and personalized consultations that resonate with potential clients. These efforts not only drive sales but also promote financial literacy and access to life insurance products in historically underserved markets.

Technology and innovation are also supporting diversity and inclusion initiatives in the life insurance sector. Digital platforms and remote work capabilities enable companies to recruit and retain agents from a wider geographic range, including those in rural or underserved areas. Virtual networking and training sessions make it easier for diverse agents to access resources and build connections within the industry. Moreover, data analytics tools can help companies identify gaps in diversity and track progress in achieving inclusion goals.

The benefits of a diverse and inclusive workforce extend beyond serving clients. Research consistently shows that diverse teams are more innovative, better at problem-solving, and more effective at decision-making. In the life insurance industry, this translates to developing creative solutions, designing products that appeal to a broader audience, and staying competitive in an increasingly globalized market.

However, challenges remain. The life insurance sector, like many industries, has historically been dominated by certain demographic groups, and overcoming entrenched biases requires sustained effort. Companies must remain committed to their diversity and inclusion goals, even when progress feels slow. Transparent reporting on diversity metrics and accountability at the leadership level are essential for maintaining momentum and fostering trust among employees.

In conclusion, promoting diversity and inclusion in the life insurance workforce is both a moral imperative and a business necessity. By attracting and retaining talent from underrepresented groups, life insurance companies can better serve an increasingly diverse client base, drive innovation, and build a more equitable industry. Efforts to create accessible career pathways, foster inclusive workplace cultures, and leverage technology are paving the way for a future where all agents, regardless of their background, can thrive and contribute meaningfully to the success of the industry. This commitment to diversity and inclusion not only strengthens the workforce but also ensures that life insurance remains relevant and accessible to all communities.

Section XIV

The Role of Life Insurance Agents in Addressing Underinsurance

How Agents Can Educate Communities About Adequate Coverage and Reduce the Protection Gap

Underinsurance is a significant issue that affects individuals, families, and communities worldwide. Many people either lack sufficient life insurance coverage or have no coverage at all, leaving them vulnerable to financial instability in the face of unexpected events. Life insurance agents play a critical role in addressing this protection gap by educating communities about the importance of adequate coverage, tailoring solutions to individual needs, and actively working to make life insurance accessible to underserved populations. By taking proactive steps, agents can ensure that more individuals and families achieve financial security and resilience.

One of the primary reasons for underinsurance is a lack of understanding about life insurance and its benefits. Many individuals are unaware of the various types of coverage available, how policies work, or the risks of being inadequately insured. Agents are uniquely positioned to bridge this knowledge gap by serving as educators within their communities. Through workshops, seminars, and one-on-one consultations, agents can demystify life insurance concepts and help clients understand the value of protecting their financial future. For example, agents can explain how life insurance not only provides for dependents in the event of a policyholder's death but also helps cover debts, final expenses, and estate taxes, or serves as a tool for wealth building and retirement planning.

To make their educational efforts more impactful, agents must tailor their messaging to the specific needs and concerns of their audience. Different communities face different financial challenges, and a one-size-fits-all approach is unlikely to resonate. For instance, in low-income communities, agents might focus on affordable term life insurance options that provide essential coverage without imposing a significant financial burden. In contrast, for higher-income families, discussions might center around policies designed for estate planning or tax efficiency. By addressing the unique circumstances of each client, agents can make life insurance more relevant and appealing.

Agents can also leverage technology to educate communities and reduce the protection gap. Digital platforms, such as social media, blogs, and webinars, enable agents to reach a broader audience and share valuable information about life insurance in an accessible format. Online tools, such as coverage calculators and comparison guides, can empower individuals to assess their needs and explore their options before engaging with an agent. Agents who embrace these technologies not only expand their reach but also position themselves as trusted advisors in a digital-first world.

Another important aspect of addressing underinsurance is overcoming common barriers to purchasing life insurance. Cost is one of the most frequently cited reasons for not having adequate coverage, but agents can help clients understand that life insurance is more affordable than many believe. By presenting flexible solutions, such as term policies with lower premiums or combination policies that provide additional benefits, agents can demonstrate that life insurance is within reach for a wide range of budgets. Agents can also educate clients about the long-term financial consequences of remaining uninsured, helping them see life insurance as an investment in their family's security rather than an expense.

Misconceptions about life insurance are another significant barrier that agents can address through education. For example, many people assume they don't need coverage if they are young, healthy, or single, or they may underestimate the amount of coverage required to protect their families adequately. Agents can dispel these myths by providing personalized assessments and explaining the potential risks of being underinsured. For instance, they can illustrate how inflation affects the real value of coverage over time or how life insurance can provide essential support for aging parents or other dependents.

Agents also play a vital role in reaching underserved and underinsured populations. Certain groups, such as minorities, immigrants, and rural communities, often face additional challenges in accessing life insurance, including language barriers, cultural misconceptions, or geographic isolation. Agents can address these challenges by building trust within these communities, offering bilingual services, and tailoring their outreach efforts to meet specific cultural or regional needs. Partnering with community organizations, churches, or local businesses can further enhance an agent's ability to connect with these populations and provide the education and resources needed to bridge the protection gap.

Proactive engagement is another strategy agents can use to address underinsurance. Instead of waiting for clients to approach them, agents can take the initiative to identify individuals or groups who may be at risk of being underinsured. For example, agents can target new parents, newlyweds, or first-time homeowners with information about the importance of life insurance in protecting their growing responsibilities. Hosting events, such as financial planning workshops or "life insurance awareness" days, can also create opportunities to educate and engage with prospective clients.

Ongoing client support is essential in ensuring that coverage remains adequate over time. Agents should conduct regular policy reviews with their clients to assess whether their needs have changed due to life events such as marriage, childbirth, or retirement. By offering these reviews as a value-added service, agents can help clients adjust their coverage as needed and avoid becoming underinsured. This long-term relationship-building fosters trust and loyalty while ensuring that clients remain financially protected.

Finally, agents can advocate for systemic changes that make life insurance more accessible and equitable. This includes collaborating with insurers to develop innovative products that address affordability and flexibility concerns or pushing for regulatory changes that simplify underwriting processes for underserved populations. Agents who participate in industry-wide initiatives to reduce the protection gap not only contribute to their communities' well-being but also enhance the reputation and inclusivity of the life insurance sector.

In conclusion, life insurance agents play a pivotal role in addressing underinsurance by educating communities, tailoring solutions to individual needs, and removing barriers to coverage. Through personalized outreach, proactive engagement, and ongoing client support, agents can help close the protection gap and ensure that more individuals and families achieve financial security. By combining expertise, empathy, and innovation, agents can transform underinsurance into an opportunity to serve their communities while building trust and value in the life insurance industry.

Section XV

Building Client Relationships: The Foundation of a Successful Life Insurance Career

A successful life insurance career is built on strong, trust-based relationships with clients. Unlike transactional sales, life insurance involves deeply personal decisions that require agents to understand their clients' financial goals, life priorities, and unique circumstances. Establishing and nurturing these relationships ensures not only initial sales but also long-term client loyalty and satisfaction. By focusing on trust-building, client retention, and delivering ongoing value, life insurance agents can create a sustainable and rewarding career while providing meaningful service to their clients.

Trust is the cornerstone of any client-agent relationship. Clients need to feel confident that their agent has their best interests at heart and is genuinely committed to helping them achieve financial security. Agents build trust by demonstrating expertise, transparency, and reliability. Expertise involves having in-depth knowledge of life insurance products and the ability to explain them clearly and confidently. Clients are more likely to trust an agent who can answer their questions thoroughly and provide tailored recommendations based on their specific needs. Transparency is equally important. Agents should disclose all relevant information about policies, including costs, benefits, and potential limitations, so clients can make informed decisions. Reliability, or consistently following through on commitments, reinforces trust over time. Whether it's returning phone calls promptly or providing regular updates, small acts of dependability can make a big difference in how clients perceive an agent's professionalism and integrity.

Personalization is another key factor in building strong client relationships. Life insurance is not a one-size-fits-all product; every client has unique goals, financial circumstances, and concerns. Agents who take the time to understand these factors and tailor their recommendations accordingly demonstrate that they value their clients as individuals. This requires active listening and empathy—skills that enable agents to uncover what truly matters to their clients. For example, a young couple might prioritize affordable term insurance to protect their growing family, while a retiree may be more interested in estate planning solutions. By aligning their advice with the client's priorities, agents can foster deeper connections and establish themselves as trusted advisors.

Client retention is just as important as attracting new clients, and it hinges on ongoing engagement and support. Life insurance is a long-term commitment, and clients need to feel that their agent is invested in their financial well-being beyond the initial policy sale. Regular check-ins are an effective way to maintain this connection. Agents can schedule annual reviews to reassess their clients' coverage needs, especially after major life events such as marriage, the birth of a child, or a career change. These reviews not only ensure that clients have adequate protection but also reinforce the agent's role as a proactive and caring partner in their financial journey.

Education is another powerful tool for retaining clients and providing long-term value. Many people find life insurance complex and intimidating, which can lead to misunderstandings or dissatisfaction. Agents who prioritize client education help demystify the process, empowering clients to make informed decisions and feel confident in their choices. This might involve explaining how policies work, addressing common misconceptions, or providing updates on new products and industry trends. Educational efforts can take various forms, including personalized consultations, newsletters, or informational webinars. By positioning themselves as knowledgeable resources, agents strengthen their relationships and build client loyalty.

Providing long-term value also means staying adaptable to clients' changing needs. As clients progress through different stages of life, their financial priorities often evolve. For instance, a policy purchased during early adulthood may no longer align with a client's goals as they approach retirement. Agents who anticipate these shifts and proactively recommend adjustments demonstrate their commitment to serving clients over the long haul. This could involve converting a term policy to a permanent one, adding riders for long-term care or critical illness coverage, or exploring cash-value options for retirement income. These personalized recommendations show clients that their agent is attuned to their needs and invested in their future.

Strong communication skills are essential for both trust-building and client retention. Effective communication involves more than just speaking clearly; it's about fostering open, two-way dialogue. Agents should encourage clients to share their concerns, ask questions, and provide feedback. This helps clients feel heard and valued while giving agents deeper insights into their needs. Active listening is particularly important, as it allows agents to pick up on subtle cues and build rapport. Additionally, agents should communicate in a way that resonates with their clients, whether that means simplifying technical jargon or using visual aids to explain complex concepts.

Building relationships also involves exceeding client expectations. Small gestures, such as sending birthday cards, congratulating clients on milestones, or checking in during difficult times, can leave a lasting impression. These actions demonstrate genuine care and help agents stand out in a competitive market. Going the extra mile creates positive experiences that clients are likely to remember and share with others, paving the way for referrals and word-of-mouth recommendations.

Agents who prioritize building relationships are also better positioned to handle challenges and objections. When trust and rapport are established, clients are more willing to have open conversations about their concerns, whether it's affordability, perceived complexity, or the timing of a purchase. Agents can use these moments as opportunities to educate, reassure, and demonstrate their commitment to finding the best solutions for the client. This collaborative approach not only resolves immediate issues but also strengthens the overall relationship.

Technology can play a supportive role in building and maintaining client relationships. Customer relationship management (CRM) systems allow agents to keep track of client interactions, preferences, and policy details, ensuring personalized and timely service. Digital communication tools, such as email newsletters and social media platforms, provide additional channels for staying connected and sharing valuable information. While technology enhances efficiency and reach, it's important for agents to balance digital interactions with personal touches, as the human element remains central to relationship-building.

In conclusion, building client relationships is the foundation of a successful life insurance career. By focusing on trust, personalization, education, and long-term support, agents can create meaningful connections that drive client loyalty and satisfaction. Strong communication, adaptability, and a genuine commitment to serving clients' best interests are key to establishing a reputation as a trusted advisor. In an industry built on trust and financial security, nurturing relationships not only ensures business success but also enables agents to make a lasting positive impact on the lives of their clients.

Section XVI

Life Insurance Agents as Educators: Simplifying Complex Products for Clients

Life insurance agents play a crucial role as educators, guiding clients through the often-overwhelming process of understanding life insurance products and their implications. For many people, life insurance policies can seem confusing or intimidating due to the technical jargon, intricate terms, and variety of options available. Agents serve as trusted guides, breaking down complex concepts into simpler, relatable terms, and empowering clients to make informed decisions that align with their financial goals. By adopting clear communication strategies, personalized approaches, and accessible tools, life insurance agents can demystify policies and foster trust, ensuring clients feel confident about their choices.

One of the most important aspects of an agent's role as an educator is translating technical language into everyday terms. Life insurance policies are filled with terminology—such as premiums, cash value, riders, and death benefits—that may be unfamiliar to the average client. Agents must be adept at explaining these concepts in ways that resonate with their audience. For instance, instead of simply stating that a term policy provides coverage for a set period, an agent might say, "This policy protects your family financially for the next 20 years, ensuring they won't face financial hardship if something happens to you during that time." This approach bridges the gap between industry jargon and the client's understanding, making the information more relatable and actionable.

Personalization is another powerful tool in the agent's educational arsenal. Every client has unique financial needs, life circumstances, and concerns, which means a one-size-fits-all explanation is rarely effective. Agents should take the time to understand their clients' goals, family dynamics, and financial situations before presenting policy options. For example, an agent might tailor their explanation of permanent life insurance by highlighting its cash value component for a client interested in building wealth, while emphasizing its stability and guaranteed payout for a client focused on leaving a legacy. Personalization ensures that clients see the relevance of life insurance to their specific needs, enhancing their engagement and confidence in the decision-making process.

Visual aids and illustrative examples are particularly helpful for simplifying complex products. Charts, graphs, and comparison tables can make it easier for clients to understand differences between policies, such as term versus permanent insurance, or the cost and benefit trade-offs of various riders. Similarly, agents can use real-life scenarios to explain how policies work in practice. For instance, they might describe how a family used a life insurance policy to pay off a mortgage or cover college tuition after the unexpected loss of a loved one. These tangible examples provide context and help clients visualize the real-world benefits of life insurance.

Education is not just about explaining products—it's also about addressing misconceptions and fears. Many clients harbor misunderstandings about life insurance, such as believing it's too expensive, unnecessary for young or single individuals, or only valuable in the event of death. Agents must proactively dispel these myths by providing accurate information and emphasizing the broader benefits of life insurance, such as income replacement, debt protection, and retirement planning. For example, agents can show clients that term life insurance is often more affordable than they assume or explain how policies with living benefits can provide financial support during a critical illness.

Storytelling is another effective technique for demystifying life insurance. Sharing real-world success stories or hypothetical scenarios allows agents to connect emotionally with clients while illustrating the practical applications of different policies. For example, an agent might recount how a term life insurance policy allowed a grieving family to remain in their home after the policyholder's passing or how a permanent life insurance policy funded a retiree's long-term care expenses. Stories like these humanize the product and demonstrate its value in relatable terms.

Agents also play a critical role in helping clients navigate the decision-making process. Choosing a life insurance policy involves evaluating multiple factors, including coverage amount, term length, premium affordability, and additional benefits. Agents can simplify this process by breaking it into manageable steps. For example, they might start by helping clients assess their financial responsibilities—such as mortgages, education expenses, or income replacement needs—before recommending a suitable coverage amount. By guiding clients through a structured decision-making process, agents reduce the stress and confusion often associated with choosing a policy.

Proactive communication and follow-up are essential components of an agent's role as an educator. Clients' needs and circumstances can change over time, whether due to marriage, the birth of a child, or changes in employment. Agents who maintain regular contact with their clients can ensure that their policies remain relevant and sufficient as these changes occur. During these check-ins, agents can provide updates on new products, explain policy options that align with the client's evolving goals, and address any lingering questions. This ongoing education fosters trust and reinforces the agent's commitment to the client's long-term financial well-being.

Technology also enhances the agent's ability to educate clients. Online tools such as coverage calculators, policy simulators, and video tutorials can complement one-on-one consultations by providing clients with interactive and accessible ways to explore their options. Digital platforms also allow agents to share resources, such as blogs, webinars, and infographics, that demystify life insurance concepts and keep clients informed about industry trends. Agents who embrace technology can extend their educational reach and ensure that clients have access to the information they need, when and where they need it.

In addition to educating individual clients, agents can take a broader approach by hosting community workshops, webinars, or financial literacy events. These initiatives allow agents to reach a wider audience and address common questions or concerns about life insurance. For example, an agent might organize a seminar on "Life Insurance 101," where they cover the basics of policy types, benefits, and how to determine coverage needs. Community education efforts not only help clients but also position the agent as a knowledgeable and approachable resource, enhancing their reputation and credibility.

Ultimately, the role of a life insurance agent as an educator is about empowering clients to make informed, confident decisions. By simplifying complex products, addressing misconceptions, and providing personalized guidance, agents help clients see the value of life insurance and understand how it fits into their broader financial goals. This educational approach builds trust, fosters long-term relationships, and ensures that clients feel supported throughout their financial journey. In an industry where trust and understanding are paramount, agents who embrace their role as educators can make a lasting impact on their clients' lives while achieving professional success.

Section XVII

Life Insurance in a Post-Pandemic World: Challenges and Opportunities for Agents

The COVID-19 pandemic brought unprecedented challenges to individuals and industries worldwide, and its impact on the life insurance sector has been profound. It reshaped client priorities, heightened awareness of financial security, and accelerated the adoption of technology, leading to a transformed landscape for life insurance agents. While the pandemic introduced challenges such as heightened mortality concerns, economic uncertainty, and shifting consumer behaviors, it also opened opportunities for agents to innovate, educate, and expand their reach. Understanding this duality is crucial for agents looking to adapt and thrive in the post-pandemic world.

One of the most significant changes brought about by the pandemic is a heightened awareness of mortality and financial vulnerability among clients. Many individuals witnessed the devastating financial impact of unexpected illness or death on families, leading to an increased interest in life insurance. Agents have seen a surge in inquiries from clients seeking protection for their loved ones and ways to mitigate financial risks during uncertain times. This growing awareness provides agents with an opportunity to educate clients about the importance of life insurance and address coverage gaps. For instance, agents can emphasize how policies can provide income replacement, cover final expenses, or support dependents in the event of a loss.

However, the pandemic also highlighted disparities in financial literacy and access to life insurance products, especially in underserved communities. Many individuals remained uninsured or underinsured due to a lack of awareness, cultural misconceptions, or financial constraints. Agents now face the challenge of bridging this protection gap by reaching out to these communities with targeted education and affordable policy options. By partnering with community organizations, leveraging digital tools, and tailoring messaging to address specific needs, agents can play a pivotal role in extending life insurance coverage to those who need it most.

Economic uncertainty during and after the pandemic has also influenced consumer behavior. Job losses, reduced incomes, and market volatility led many clients to reevaluate their financial priorities. For some, this meant postponing or downsizing life insurance purchases, while others sought affordable solutions like term life insurance to ensure basic protection. Agents have had to navigate these shifting priorities by offering flexible, cost-effective options and helping clients understand the long-term value of life insurance. The ability to present life insurance as a financial safety net rather than an additional expense has become a critical skill for agents in the post-pandemic landscape.

The pandemic also accelerated the digital transformation of the life insurance industry. Social distancing measures and lockdowns forced agents and insurers to adapt quickly to remote communication and digital processes. Virtual consultations, online policy applications, and e-signatures became the norm, making life insurance more accessible and convenient for clients. This shift has provided agents with new tools to engage with clients, but it also introduced challenges in building trust and rapport in a virtual environment. Agents must strike a balance between leveraging digital technologies and maintaining the personal touch that is crucial in life insurance sales.

The increased reliance on technology has also expanded opportunities for data-driven decision-making and personalized service. Digital platforms enable agents to analyze client data, identify coverage needs, and recommend tailored solutions. For example, predictive analytics can help agents determine which clients are most likely to benefit from specific policies or identify potential gaps in coverage. Agents who embrace these technologies can provide more precise and efficient service, enhancing client satisfaction and retention.

The pandemic has reshaped not only client priorities but also the types of products that are in demand. Hybrid policies that combine life insurance with other benefits, such as long-term care or critical illness coverage, have gained popularity as clients seek comprehensive protection. Similarly, policies with living benefits, which allow policyholders to access a portion of the death benefit during their lifetime, have become more appealing in light of the healthcare challenges highlighted by the pandemic. Agents must stay informed about these emerging products and educate clients on their advantages to meet evolving needs.

Another important shift in the post-pandemic world is the growing emphasis on health and wellness. Clients are increasingly interested in policies that reward healthy behaviors, such as wearable tech integration or wellness programs that offer premium discounts. Agents can capitalize on this trend by highlighting policies that incentivize healthier lifestyles and explaining how these features align with broader health and financial goals.

Despite the opportunities, agents face ongoing challenges in the post-pandemic environment. One significant hurdle is addressing clients' skepticism or misinformation about life insurance. The pandemic revealed widespread misconceptions about coverage, such as the belief that life insurance policies would not pay out for COVID-related deaths. Agents must prioritize clear communication and education to dispel myths and build trust with clients. Transparency about policy terms, exclusions, and benefits is essential for fostering confidence in the value of life insurance.

The psychological impact of the pandemic also presents challenges for agents. Clients who experienced loss or financial hardship may approach life insurance discussions with heightened anxiety or resistance. Agents need to demonstrate empathy, patience, and sensitivity when addressing these concerns. Establishing a supportive and non-judgmental environment can help clients feel more comfortable discussing their needs and exploring solutions.

The pandemic has also underscored the importance of resilience and adaptability for life insurance agents. As the industry continues to evolve, agents must remain proactive in updating their knowledge, embracing new technologies, and refining their communication skills. Continuing education and professional development will be key to staying relevant and effective in meeting clients' needs.

In conclusion, the post-pandemic world presents both challenges and opportunities for life insurance agents. The heightened awareness of financial vulnerability, the shift toward digital engagement, and the evolving demand for innovative products create a dynamic environment that requires agents to adapt and innovate. By focusing on education, empathy, and personalization, agents can help clients navigate their new priorities and achieve financial security. In doing so, they not only contribute to the well-being of their clients but also strengthen their own careers in a rapidly changing industry.

Section XVIII

Group Life Insurance Sales: Strategies for Agents in Corporate Markets

Approaches for Selling Life Insurance to Businesses and Organizations for Employee Benefits

Group life insurance is a vital component of employee benefits packages, offering protection to employees and their families while enhancing the employer's ability to attract and retain talent. For life insurance agents, selling group life insurance to businesses and organizations presents a unique opportunity to secure high-volume sales and establish long-term relationships with corporate clients. Success in this market requires a strategic approach that combines understanding corporate needs, demonstrating the value of group life insurance, and building trust with decision-makers. By adopting tailored strategies, agents can effectively navigate the corporate market and maximize their impact.

To sell group life insurance to businesses, agents must first understand the corporate client's perspective. Employers seek benefits packages that align with their workforce's needs and support their organizational goals. Group life insurance is particularly attractive because it is cost-effective, provides employees with a sense of financial security, and demonstrates the employer's commitment to their well-being. Agents must position group life insurance as an integral part of the employer's overall benefits strategy, emphasizing its role in fostering employee loyalty, improving morale, and enhancing the company's competitive edge in the job market.

The initial step in approaching a corporate client is conducting thorough research to understand their business, workforce demographics, and existing benefits offerings. For example, an agent working with a technology startup might focus on the need to attract and retain young talent, while a proposal for a manufacturing company might emphasize coverage for a workforce with diverse family responsibilities. Tailoring the pitch to the organization's specific needs ensures relevance and demonstrates the agent's dedication to providing customized solutions.

When presenting group life insurance to businesses, agents must articulate its value clearly and compellingly. This involves explaining how group policies differ from individual coverage, highlighting benefits such as simplified underwriting, lower premiums, and the ability to extend coverage to all employees regardless of pre-existing conditions. Agents should also underscore the flexibility of group plans, which can be structured to include basic coverage funded by the employer, as well as voluntary supplemental options that employees can purchase at their discretion. This flexibility allows businesses to offer robust benefits without significantly increasing costs.

Cost is a major consideration for corporate clients, and agents must address it effectively. Employers often operate within tight budgets and demonstrating the affordability of group life insurance is critical. Agents can provide detailed cost analyses, including the employer's contribution per employee and the potential return on investment in terms of employee satisfaction and retention. Offering multiple plan options at varying price points allows employers to choose a solution that fits their budget while meeting their workforce's needs. Agents can also highlight the tax advantages of group life insurance for businesses, further enhancing its appeal.

Building trust with decision-makers is essential for closing group life insurance sales. Agents must establish credibility by demonstrating their expertise and understanding of the corporate market. This includes being well-versed in regulatory requirements, such as compliance with the Employee Retirement Income Security Act (ERISA) or other applicable laws, and addressing any legal concerns the employer might have. Additionally, agents should present data-driven insights, such as industry benchmarks and employee surveys, to support their recommendations. Providing case studies or testimonials from similar businesses that have successfully implemented group life insurance plans can further reinforce trust.

Effective communication with multiple stakeholders is another critical aspect of selling group life insurance. In many organizations, the decision-making process involves various parties, including human resources (HR), finance, and senior management. Agents must tailor their messaging to address the priorities of each stakeholder. For example, HR professionals may focus on employee satisfaction and retention, while financial officers may prioritize cost-effectiveness and budget alignment. Agents who can address the concerns of all stakeholders and present a cohesive value proposition are more likely to succeed.

Engaging employees is also a key component of group life insurance sales. Even after a company decides to offer a group plan, employees must understand and appreciate its value to take full advantage of the benefits. Agents can support employers by providing educational materials, hosting enrollment meetings, and offering one-on-one consultations with employees to explain the plan's features. This proactive engagement not only boosts employee participation but also strengthens the agent's relationship with the corporate client.

Technology plays an increasingly important role in group life insurance sales. Digital tools and platforms streamline the enrollment process, making it easier for employers to manage and for employees to access their benefits. Agents who offer user-friendly solutions, such as online portals for policy administration or mobile apps for employees to view their coverage, can differentiate themselves from competitors. These tools also enable agents to track enrollment data and provide ongoing support, ensuring a seamless experience for the client.

Agents can further enhance their value by offering ancillary services or bundling group life insurance with other products, such as health insurance, disability coverage, or retirement planning services. This comprehensive approach allows agents to become a one-stop solution for the employer's benefits needs, increasing the likelihood of securing long-term contracts and repeat business.

Networking and relationship-building are crucial for success in the corporate market. Agents should actively engage with industry associations, attend HR and benefits conferences, and participate in local business networking events to connect with potential clients. Establishing a presence in these spaces not only helps agents identify leads but also positions them as knowledgeable and trusted professionals in the employee benefits field.

In conclusion, selling group life insurance in the corporate market requires a strategic and client-focused approach. By understanding the needs of businesses, tailoring solutions to specific challenges, and building strong relationships with decision-makers, agents can effectively position group life insurance as an essential component of employee benefits packages. The combination of affordability, flexibility, and value makes group life insurance an attractive proposition for employers, while proactive communication, education, and technology integration ensure a positive experience for both businesses and their employees. By adopting these strategies, agents can expand their client base, secure long-term partnerships, and thrive in the competitive corporate market.

Section XIX

Navigating Regulatory Changes as a Life Insurance Agent

Keeping Up with Changing Laws and Regulations and Their Impact on Policy Sales and Compliance

The life insurance industry operates within a highly regulated environment, where laws and regulations are constantly evolving to address economic shifts, technological advancements, and consumer protection concerns. For life insurance agents, staying informed about regulatory changes is essential to maintaining compliance, preserving client trust, and ensuring seamless policy sales. Navigating these changes requires a proactive approach, a commitment to ongoing education, and a clear understanding of how new rules impact both business practices and client relationships. By keeping pace with regulatory updates and adapting to their implications, agents can remain competitive and deliver ethical, high-quality service.

One of the most significant challenges for life insurance agents is the dynamic nature of industry regulations. Changes may occur at the federal, state, or local level, affecting areas such as licensing requirements, product offerings, marketing practices, and data privacy standards. For example, states may introduce new continuing education mandates, or federal legislation may revise tax laws that impact life insurance policies. Additionally, regulations like the Gramm-Leach-Bliley Act (GLBA) or state-specific consumer protection laws often require agents to adjust their business practices to ensure compliance with privacy and disclosure standards.

Staying ahead of these changes involves continuous learning and active engagement with industry resources. Agents must dedicate time to studying regulatory updates from agencies such as state insurance departments, the National Association of Insurance Commissioners (NAIC), and other governing bodies. Subscribing to industry publications, attending compliance webinars, and participating in professional associations provide valuable insights into emerging rules and best practices for adapting to them. Agents who prioritize ongoing education not only ensure compliance but also position themselves as knowledgeable professionals who can confidently guide clients through the complexities of life insurance.

Regulatory changes can significantly impact the products agents sell and how they present these products to clients. For instance, updates to tax laws may alter the advantages of certain life insurance policies, such as the tax-deferred growth of cash value in permanent life insurance. Agents must stay informed about these changes to accurately convey the benefits and limitations of policies to clients. Similarly, new rules governing product disclosures may require agents to update their sales materials and communication strategies to ensure transparency and compliance.

Data privacy and cybersecurity regulations are increasingly relevant to life insurance agents in an era of digital transformation. Laws such as the California Consumer Privacy Act (CCPA) or the General Data Protection Regulation (GDPR) impose strict requirements on how agents collect, store, and share client information. Noncompliance with these rules can result in severe penalties and damage to an agent's reputation. To navigate these challenges, agents must adopt secure data management practices, implement robust cybersecurity measures, and educate themselves on the legal obligations surrounding client data. Providing clear privacy policies and obtaining explicit consent from clients when handling their information are critical steps in maintaining compliance.

Regulatory changes also affect the marketing and advertising practices of life insurance agents. For example, agents must adhere to rules that govern the use of testimonials, endorsements, and claims in promotional materials. Misleading or exaggerated statements can lead to legal repercussions and loss of licensure. Staying compliant requires agents to carefully review marketing content, ensure all claims are substantiated, and avoid deceptive practices. Additionally, agents must be aware of rules related to social media and digital advertising, which are becoming increasingly common platforms for reaching clients.

Navigating regulatory changes is not only about compliance but also about building trust with clients. Clients expect their agents to act ethically and transparently, providing accurate information and safeguarding their interests. Agents who proactively address regulatory updates in client interactions demonstrate professionalism and a commitment to doing what is right. For instance, an agent might explain how a new law affects an existing policy or highlight how compliance measures protect the client's privacy and security. These efforts build confidence and foster long-term client relationships.

Collaboration with compliance teams and legal professionals is another critical aspect of navigating regulatory changes. Many insurance companies have dedicated compliance departments that provide agents with guidance on implementing new rules and avoiding common pitfalls. Agents should actively seek out this support, attending training sessions and consulting with compliance officers as needed. For independent agents, forming partnerships with legal advisors or third-party compliance consultants can help ensure adherence to complex regulations and reduce the risk of errors.

Regulatory changes also present opportunities for agents to differentiate themselves in the market. By staying informed and adaptable, agents can position themselves as experts who add value beyond policy sales. For example, an agent who thoroughly understands the implications of recent tax law changes can provide clients with insights on how to optimize their coverage for estate planning or retirement. Similarly, agents who demonstrate fluency in data privacy regulations can reassure clients that their information is being handled securely and responsibly.

One of the most effective ways for agents to manage regulatory changes is through technology. Compliance management software, for instance, helps agents track updates, monitor business practices, and generate reports to demonstrate adherence to legal standards. Digital tools also facilitate secure communication and record-keeping, ensuring that agents meet documentation requirements. By leveraging technology, agents can streamline compliance efforts and focus more on serving their clients.

Despite the challenges, navigating regulatory changes is ultimately an opportunity for growth and professional development. Agents who embrace these changes as part of their role deepen their expertise, enhance their credibility, and strengthen their client relationships. By staying informed, collaborating with compliance resources, and adopting innovative practices, agents can turn regulatory complexities into a competitive advantage.

In conclusion, navigating regulatory changes is an integral part of being a life insurance agent. The ability to stay informed, adapt to new rules, and maintain compliance not only protects the agent's business but also builds trust with clients and ensures the delivery of ethical, high-quality service. In a rapidly evolving industry, agents who prioritize continuous learning, leverage technology, and collaborate with compliance professionals will be well-positioned to succeed while meeting the highest standards of integrity and professionalism.

Section XX

The Future of Life Insurance Sales: Trends Shaping the Agent's Role

Examining Where the Industry Is Headed and How Agents Can Stay Relevant

The life insurance industry is undergoing a profound transformation driven by advancements in technology, shifting consumer preferences, and evolving market dynamics. These changes are redefining the role of life insurance agents, creating both challenges and opportunities. As the industry moves forward, agents must adapt to new trends, adopt innovative strategies, and embrace professional growth to remain relevant and effective in meeting the needs of their clients. Understanding these emerging trends and their implications is crucial for agents looking to thrive in the future of life insurance sales.

One of the most significant trends shaping the industry is the increasing digitization of life insurance sales and services. Digital platforms, AI-driven tools, and online customer portals are revolutionizing how clients interact with life insurance products. The rise of InsurTech companies has introduced seamless, direct-to-consumer platforms that allow clients to compare policies, get quotes, and purchase coverage online with minimal agent involvement. While this shift poses challenges to traditional agent-client interactions, it also provides opportunities for agents to leverage technology to enhance their services. Agents who embrace digital tools can streamline processes, such as policy applications and underwriting, while focusing their efforts on providing personalized advice and building relationships.

Another major trend is the growing demand for personalized and flexible life insurance solutions. Modern consumers expect tailored products that adapt to their unique life circumstances and financial goals. This shift is particularly evident among younger generations, who prioritize customization and value in their purchasing decisions. Agents must adapt by deepening their understanding of client needs and recommending policies that offer adjustable coverage, hybrid benefits, or value-added features like health and wellness incentives. Personalized consultations and financial planning services will become key differentiators for agents in a market where customization is paramount.

The integration of data analytics and artificial intelligence (AI) is also transforming the life insurance landscape. Predictive analytics enables insurers and agents to identify trends, assess risks, and recommend suitable policies with greater precision. AI-powered tools can streamline underwriting, automate routine tasks, and provide actionable insights into client behavior. For agents, this means a shift toward becoming data-driven advisors who leverage insights to create value for their clients. Agents who invest in understanding and utilizing these technologies will be better positioned to offer informed, timely, and impactful recommendations.

Shifting demographic trends are another factor shaping the future of life insurance sales. As populations become more diverse, agents must adapt their strategies to meet the needs of multicultural markets. This includes offering culturally relevant solutions, addressing unique financial priorities, and building trust with clients from various backgrounds. Agents who invest in cultural competency and develop inclusive practices will be better equipped to serve a broader range of clients, fostering trust and loyalty in underrepresented communities.

Sustainability and social responsibility are also influencing the life insurance industry. Consumers are increasingly looking for companies and professionals who align with their values, including environmental stewardship and ethical business practices. Insurers are responding by developing policies tied to sustainability initiatives, such as investments in green projects or carbon offset programs. Agents can position themselves as socially conscious advisors by promoting these products and demonstrating a commitment to positive societal impact. This approach not only appeals to environmentally aware clients but also enhances the agent's reputation as a forward-thinking professional.

The rise of hybrid work models and virtual client interactions has reshaped how agents conduct business. The COVID-19 pandemic accelerated the adoption of remote communication tools, such as video conferencing and digital document sharing, making them an integral part of the agent-client relationship. While face-to-face meetings remain valuable, agents must become proficient in virtual engagement to connect with clients effectively, regardless of geographic location. Offering flexible communication options ensures that clients feel supported and valued, enhancing the overall customer experience.

Financial literacy education is becoming an increasingly important aspect of the agent's role. Many clients, particularly younger generations, lack a thorough understanding of life insurance and its benefits. Agents who position themselves as educators can bridge this knowledge gap, empowering clients to make informed decisions. This involves simplifying complex concepts, offering resources like webinars or articles, and providing ongoing support throughout the policy lifecycle. By prioritizing education, agents build trust and establish themselves as indispensable partners in their clients' financial journeys.

The emergence of holistic financial planning is blurring the lines between traditional life insurance sales and broader advisory services. Clients are seeking comprehensive solutions that integrate life insurance with retirement planning, estate management, and investment strategies. This trend presents an opportunity for agents to expand their expertise and offer value-added services that address the full spectrum of their clients' financial needs. Agents who pursue advanced certifications, such as the Certified Financial Planner (CFP) or Chartered Life Underwriter (CLU) designations, can differentiate themselves in this evolving market.

Ethical considerations and compliance will continue to play a critical role in shaping the agent's responsibilities. As regulations evolve to enhance consumer protection and ensure transparency, agents must stay informed about legal requirements and industry standards. This includes understanding privacy laws, avoiding deceptive sales practices, and adhering to suitability standards when recommending policies. By prioritizing ethics and compliance, agents not only safeguard their careers but also build lasting trust with their clients.

Resilience and adaptability are essential traits for agents navigating the future of life insurance sales. The industry's rapid evolution demands a commitment to lifelong learning and professional development. Agents must stay informed about emerging trends, continuously refine their skills, and be willing to embrace change. Participating in workshops, joining industry associations, and leveraging mentorship opportunities can help agents stay ahead of the curve and maintain their relevance in a competitive market.

In conclusion, the future of life insurance sales is marked by significant change, driven by technology, shifting consumer expectations, and evolving market dynamics. For agents, staying relevant requires a proactive approach that combines innovation, education, and adaptability. By embracing digital transformation, personalizing their services, and expanding their expertise, agents can navigate these trends successfully and provide lasting value to their clients. In a rapidly changing industry, agents who prioritize trust, education, and ethical practices will not only remain relevant but also thrive as leaders in the future of life insurance sales.

PART THREE

Section XXII

Why?

The Agent's "Why" for Doing Insurance Business

An insurance agent's **"why"** is the core purpose and motivation behind their work in the insurance business. It goes beyond earning a living or achieving sales targets—it is rooted in the deeper meaning of what they do and the value they bring to clients, families, and communities. Understanding and embracing this **"why"** helps agents stay motivated, build meaningful relationships, and create lasting impacts on the lives of others.

At its core, the **"why"** for many agents revolves around **helping people achieve financial security and peace of mind.** Life is unpredictable, and unforeseen events—such as illness, accidents, or the loss of a loved one—can bring emotional and financial hardship. Insurance agents play a critical role in mitigating these risks by providing clients with products that protect their families, safeguard their assets, and ensure financial stability in times of crisis. Agents often take pride in knowing that the policies they sell can prevent families from losing their homes, cover critical medical expenses, or fund a child's education after the loss of a parent.

Another powerful motivator for agents is the opportunity to **educate and empower clients.** Many people lack a clear understanding of how insurance works, leaving them underinsured or uninsured. Agents act as educators, breaking down complex products into simple, relatable terms and helping clients make informed decisions. By filling this knowledge gap, agents enable individuals to take control of their financial futures and feel confident about their plans for the unexpected.

For some agents, the "**why**" stems from a **desire to make a difference in their communities.** Selling insurance is not just about individual policies; it's about contributing to the greater good by fostering resilience and stability within society. By ensuring that families, businesses, and organizations are adequately protected, agents play a role in strengthening the fabric of their communities. This sense of purpose is especially significant during times of crisis, such as natural disasters or pandemics, when insurance becomes a lifeline for many.

The "**why**" is also deeply personal for many agents, often tied to their own experiences. Some enter the insurance business because they have witnessed firsthand the devastating impact of being uninsured or underinsured. Others may have been inspired by a positive experience with an insurance policy that provided much-needed support during a difficult time. These personal connections to the importance of insurance fuel agents' passion and commitment to their work.

In addition to serving others, the **"why"** for many agents includes the **opportunity for personal growth and success.** The insurance business rewards perseverance, skill, and empathy, offering agents the chance to build their careers, achieve financial independence, and develop professionally. For entrepreneurial-minded individuals, insurance provides the flexibility to create their own schedules, build their own client base, and shape their own success. This autonomy and potential for growth align with many agents' aspirations for financial and personal fulfillment.

Lastly, the "why" is often tied to the **relationships agents build with their clients.** Insurance agents are more than just salespeople; they are trusted advisors and, often, lifelong partners in their clients' financial journeys. By taking the time to understand their clients' needs, goals, and concerns, agents forge meaningful connections that extend beyond transactions. These relationships provide a sense of purpose and satisfaction that comes from knowing they have made a difference in their clients' lives.

In summary, the "why" for doing insurance business varies among agents but is universally grounded in service, impact, and growth. It is about helping people navigate uncertainty, empowering them with knowledge, and creating a positive ripple effect in their lives and communities. For agents, this "why" serves as both a compass and a source of inspiration, driving their commitment to excellence and reinforcing the importance of their work in an ever-changing world.

Section XXIII

What?

Define your vision, mission, goals, and objectives.

An insurance agent's vision, mission, goals, and objectives serve as a roadmap for their professional journey, defining their purpose, aspirations, and strategies for achieving success. These elements not only guide the agent's actions but also shape how they serve clients, grow their business, and contribute to the broader insurance industry. To create a clear and actionable framework, it's important to understand each term, their differences, and how they work together.

Vision

A vision is the long-term aspiration or ultimate purpose that inspires an insurance agent's work. It answers the question: **"What do I want to achieve in the long run?"** A vision provides a sense of direction and reflects the agent's ideal future for their career and the impact they hope to make on their clients and community.

Definition
The vision is a forward-looking statement that describes what the agent aims to accomplish in

the future, often focusing on the broader impact of their work.

Example

An insurance agent's vision might be:
To create a financially secure and informed community where every family has access to adequate protection and peace of mind.

Key Characteristics

⇒ Long-term and aspirational
⇒ Broad and overarching
⇒ Focuses on the ultimate impact

Mission

The mission defines the agent's core purpose and day-to-day activities. It answers the question: **"Why do I do what I do, and how do I achieve it?"** A mission focuses on the present and outlines the actions the agent takes to fulfill their vision.

Definition

The mission is a statement that articulates the agent's purpose, the services they provide, and the approach they take to deliver value to clients.

Example

An insurance agent's mission might be:

To provide personalized life insurance solutions, educate clients about financial planning, and build lasting relationships based on trust and integrity.

Key Characteristics

⇒ Actionable and present-focused
⇒ Defines how the agent serves clients
⇒ Connects daily actions to long-term aspirations

Goals

Goals are broad, measurable outcomes that help the agent progress toward their vision. They answer the question: **"What specific results do I want to achieve?"** Goals provide focus and help the agent prioritize their efforts.

Definition

Goals are overarching achievements or milestones that align with the agent's vision and mission.

⇒ **Example**
   An insurance agent's goals might include:
⇒ Expanding their client base by 20% within the next year.
⇒ Becoming a top-performing agent in their region within five years.

Key Characteristics

⇒ Broad and medium-to-long-term

⇒ Measurable but not highly detailed

⇒ Focused on outcomes

Objectives

Objectives are specific, actionable steps that contribute to achieving goals. They answer the question: **"What tasks or activities must I complete to meet my goals?"** Objectives break goals into smaller, manageable actions.

Definition

Objectives are precise, time-bound actions or targets that directly support the achievement of a goal.

Example

If the agent's goal is to expand their client base by 20% within a year, their objectives might be:

⇒ Schedule five client consultations per week.

⇒ Host a financial literacy workshop every month.

⇒ Launch a social media campaign targeting new leads within the next three months.

Key Characteristics

⇒ Specific and time-bound

⇒ Highly actionable and detailed

⇒ Focused on tasks

Differences Between Vision and Mission

Focus

Vision is future-oriented and aspirational, focusing on what the agent hopes to achieve in the long term.

Mission is present-focused and practical, outlining how the agent operates to achieve the vision.

Scope

⇒ Vision is broad and idealistic.

⇒ Mission is more specific, and action driven.

Example in Context

Vision: *To ensure every individual in my community is financially protected.*

Mission: *To offer accessible and personalized life insurance products and build trust with every client I serve.*

Differences Between Goals and Objectives

Scope

⇒ Goals are broader, focusing on desired outcomes or achievements.

⇒ Objectives are narrower, specifying actionable steps to reach those goals.

Time Frame

⇒ Goals often span medium to long terms (months or years).

⇒ Objectives are short-term and specific, often tied to daily or weekly actions.

Example in Context

Goal: *Increase revenue by 25% in the next year.*

Objective: *Sell five new policies each month by scheduling 10 client meetings per week.*

Define Your Vision, Mission, Goals, and Objectives

Vision
To build a financially empowered society where every family and individual has access to personalized insurance solutions for long-term security.

Mission
To educate clients about the value of life insurance, provide

tailored financial protection plans, and offer exceptional customer service that fosters trust and loyalty.

Goals

⇒ Achieve recognition as a leading life insurance advisor in the local market within five years.

⇒ Grow annual revenue by 30% by expanding client outreach and upselling products.

⇒ Build a network of 100 satisfied long-term clients by the end of the third year.

Objectives

⇒ Schedule and complete 20 client consultations per month.

⇒ Attend two professional development workshops every quarter to refine sales techniques.

⇒ Launch a targeted marketing campaign on social media within three months to attract younger clients.

⇒ Follow up with every client annually to reassess and adjust their policies.

By defining vision, mission, goals, and objectives, agents establish a clear framework for success. The vision inspires and guides long-term aspirations, the mission reflects daily purpose, goals set measurable milestones, and objectives provide actionable steps to achieve those goals. Together, these elements ensure that agents remain focused, motivated, and effective in their work, benefiting both their clients and their professional growth.

Section XXIV

How? Learn actionable strategies to achieve success and navigate challenges.

Success in the insurance industry requires a blend of strategic planning, adaptability, and consistent execution. To thrive in this competitive field, agents must adopt actionable strategies that enable them to achieve their goals, overcome obstacles, and deliver value to their clients. These strategies should be focused on building relationships, enhancing expertise, leveraging technology, and maintaining resilience in the face of challenges.

The first step to achieving success is setting clear and measurable objectives. This involves breaking down long-term goals into smaller, actionable tasks that can be completed on a daily, weekly, or monthly basis. For example, if an agent aims to expand their client base, actionable strategies might include scheduling a specific number of consultations each week, hosting informational webinars to attract new leads, or creating a referral program to encourage existing clients to recommend their services. By focusing on specific actions, agents can create a roadmap that makes larger goals feel more attainable.

Another essential strategy is continuous learning and professional development. The insurance industry is constantly evolving due to regulatory changes, emerging technologies, and shifting consumer preferences. To stay ahead, agents must invest in their knowledge and skills by attending industry conferences, participating in workshops, earning advanced certifications, or staying updated on new product offerings. For instance, learning about hybrid policies that combine life insurance with long-term care benefits or understanding the latest in predictive analytics can help agents meet client needs more effectively. Staying informed not only enhances an agent's ability to serve their clients but also builds credibility and trust in their expertise.

Building and nurturing relationships is another cornerstone of success. Insurance is a people-centric business, and agents must prioritize trust and connection in their interactions. This involves listening to clients' concerns, tailoring solutions to their unique circumstances, and providing ongoing support throughout the life of the policy. Strong relationships also create opportunities for referrals and repeat business, as satisfied clients are more likely to recommend an agent to their family and friends. To cultivate these relationships, agents should adopt a customer-first mindset, ensuring they communicate regularly, address questions promptly, and show genuine care for their clients' financial well-being.

Leveraging technology is a critical strategy for navigating challenges and enhancing efficiency. Digital tools such as customer relationship management (CRM) systems help agents organize client information, track interactions, and automate follow-ups, enabling them to manage their workload more effectively. Virtual meeting platforms and online policy applications make it easier to connect with clients regardless of location, while data analytics tools provide insights into client preferences and purchasing behaviors. For example, an agent might use predictive analytics to identify clients who are likely to need additional coverage or to optimize marketing campaigns. Embracing technology allows agents to focus on building relationships and delivering personalized service while streamlining administrative tasks.

Resilience and adaptability are essential for overcoming challenges. The insurance business can be unpredictable, with fluctuations in market conditions, regulatory changes, and evolving client expectations. Agents must be prepared to adjust their strategies and remain focused on their goals even when faced with setbacks. This might mean reevaluating their marketing approach, learning to work effectively in a virtual environment, or finding creative solutions to meet clients' needs in difficult circumstances. Resilience also involves maintaining a positive attitude and staying motivated, which can be achieved through regular goal setting, celebrating small successes, and seeking support from mentors or peers.

Effective communication is another key strategy for navigating challenges. Agents must be able to clearly explain complex insurance concepts, address client concerns, and demonstrate the value of their services. Strong communication builds trust and ensures that clients feel confident in their decisions. Additionally, proactive communication can help agents anticipate and address potential issues before they become problems. For instance, an agent might check in with clients during times of economic uncertainty to reassess their coverage and offer guidance on how to maintain financial security.

Time management and organization are also critical for success. With numerous responsibilities, including client consultations, policy management, and professional development, agents must prioritize their tasks and allocate their time effectively. Creating a structured schedule, setting deadlines for objectives, and using productivity tools can help agents stay on track and avoid feeling overwhelmed. For example, dedicating specific hours each week to prospecting new clients or following up with existing ones ensures that these essential activities don't get overlooked.

Lastly, embracing a growth mindset is vital for long-term success. This means viewing challenges as opportunities to learn and improve rather than as obstacles. Agents with a growth mindset are more likely to seek feedback, take calculated risks, and persevere through difficulties. For instance, an agent who experiences a slow sales period might use the time to refine their skills, expand their network, or explore new markets. This proactive approach not only helps agents navigate challenges but also positions them for continued success.

In summary, achieving success and overcoming challenges in the insurance industry requires a combination of actionable strategies. By setting clear objectives, investing in professional development, building strong relationships, leveraging technology, and maintaining resilience, agents can create a foundation for sustained growth and impact. These strategies enable agents to navigate the complexities of their field while providing exceptional service to their clients, ensuring both personal fulfillment and professional success.

Section XXV

Who?
(Follow **Who** Know Road)

Understand the value of mentorship and the importance of being coachable.

In the journey toward success, the question of "Who?" is vital—who do you turn to for guidance, who can help you grow, and who exemplifies the path you want to follow? The value of mentorship and the importance of being coachable cannot be overstated in any career, especially in a field as dynamic and relationship driven as life insurance. The African proverb "Follow who know road" perfectly encapsulates this idea. It suggests that to navigate uncharted territories and avoid pitfalls, one should follow someone who has already traveled the path successfully. This wisdom applies not just to life insurance but to any pursuit that requires knowledge, skill, and perseverance.

Mentorship is one of the most powerful tools for growth. A mentor serves as a guide, offering advice, sharing experiences, and providing encouragement. In the insurance business, where success is often built on relationships, trust, and strategy, having a mentor who understands the industry can accelerate an agent's progress. A mentor who "knows the road" brings invaluable insights, helping you avoid mistakes they may have encountered and offering shortcuts to success based on their expertise. They can teach you how to handle objections, close sales, manage client relationships, and adapt to industry changes—all essential skills for a thriving career.

The phrase **Follow who know road** emphasizes the importance of choosing the right mentor. Not every successful person can be a great guide, and not every guide is equipped to help you reach your specific goals. It's crucial to identify mentors who align with your values, understand your aspirations, and have a proven track record in the areas you wish to excel. For instance, if your goal is to specialize in group life insurance sales, seeking a mentor who has excelled in that niche will provide targeted guidance that general advice cannot.

Being coachable is just as important as having a mentor. The best mentorship in the world is wasted if you are not open to learning, adapting, and applying what you are taught. Being coachable means listening actively, embracing constructive feedback, and having the humility to acknowledge that you don't know everything. It requires a willingness to step out of your comfort zone, challenge your assumptions, and implement strategies that may feel unfamiliar at first. "Follow who know road" also implies trust—trusting your mentor's guidance even when it challenges your instincts. This trust allows you to grow, learn from their wisdom, and avoid unnecessary detours on your journey.

A great example of this principle is when new agents enter the life insurance business. The industry can be overwhelming, with its complex products, sales strategies, and regulatory requirements. Agents who actively seek mentorship and remain open to guidance are more likely to find their footing and succeed. For instance, a mentor might teach a new agent how to identify high-potential leads or explain the nuances of tailoring policies to different client needs. By trusting and implementing this advice, the agent can avoid common pitfalls, build confidence, and see results more quickly.

Mentorship also extends beyond direct, one-on-one relationships. Following **who know road** can mean learning from industry leaders through books, seminars, podcasts, or training programs. Many successful individuals share their expertise and experiences in ways that can inspire and guide others. By seeking out and absorbing this knowledge, you can broaden your understanding of the road ahead and adopt proven strategies for success.

In addition to benefiting from mentorship, there is immense value in eventually becoming a mentor yourself. Sharing your journey with others, offering guidance, and helping them succeed not only strengthens the profession but also reinforces your own knowledge and skills. The cycle of mentorship—receiving guidance and then passing it on—creates a community of growth and mutual support, ensuring that the lessons learned by one generation of agents benefit those who follow.

Ultimately, the concept of "Follow who know road" is about humility, wisdom, and action. It reminds us that success is rarely achieved in isolation and that seeking guidance from those who have already navigated similar challenges is both practical and empowering. By valuing mentorship and being coachable, you position yourself to learn from the experiences of others, avoid unnecessary mistakes, and progress more confidently toward your goals. In life insurance and beyond, knowing who to follow and being willing to learn are among the most valuable traits an aspiring professional can possess.

Section XXVI

Where?

Identify the resources available to grow your business.

In any profession, and especially in life insurance, knowing "where" to find the resources that fuel growth is as important as the strategies and skills you employ. The "where" encompasses the places, tools, and opportunities that empower life insurance agents to expand their businesses, reach new clients, refine their expertise, and achieve sustainable success. By identifying and leveraging these resources, agents can turn challenges into opportunities and set the stage for consistent growth.

The first "where" lies within **professional networks and industry associations.** These organizations offer a wealth of resources, including training programs, networking events, and mentorship opportunities. Joining groups such as the National Association of Insurance and Financial Advisors (NAIFA) or regional insurance boards can connect you with seasoned professionals who share valuable insights and strategies. These networks often host conferences and workshops that provide updates on industry trends, regulatory changes, and innovative sales techniques. By actively participating, agents gain access to a community of peers who can offer support, referrals, and collaboration opportunities.

Another key resource is **continuing education and certification programs.** The life insurance industry evolves constantly, with new products, technologies, and regulations shaping the market. Agents who invest in their education remain competitive by staying informed and skilled. Online platforms, universities, and professional organizations offer courses on topics such as advanced insurance products, estate planning, and financial advisory practices. Obtaining certifications like the Chartered Life Underwriter (CLU) or Certified Financial Planner (CFP) not only enhances an agent's expertise but also elevates their credibility in the eyes of clients.

The rise of **technology and digital tools** has revolutionized the way agents operate. Customer relationship management (CRM) software, for instance, enables agents to manage client information, track interactions, and automate follow-ups, ensuring a more efficient and personalized approach to client service. Platforms like HubSpot, Salesforce, or insurance-specific tools such as Agency Bloc helps agents streamline their workflows and focus more on building relationships. Additionally, social media platforms and digital marketing tools provide powerful avenues for reaching and engaging potential clients. Agents can use Facebook, LinkedIn, or Instagram to share educational content, promote their services, and connect with a broader audience.

Agents should also explore **community-based resources.** Local chambers of commerce, small business development centers, and nonprofit organizations often provide valuable support for growing businesses. These resources can help agents develop marketing strategies, improve their sales techniques, and connect with local businesses and community leaders. For example, an agent might partner with a local small business to offer group life insurance or collaborate with a community organization to host a financial literacy workshop. These connections not only enhance visibility but also build trust within the community.

Leveraging **insurer partnerships** is another critical resource. Insurance companies often provide agents with training, marketing materials, and support systems designed to help them succeed. These resources may include product guides, co-branded marketing campaigns, or access to underwriting experts who can assist with complex cases. Some insurers even offer lead generation programs or online portals that simplify policy applications and claims processing. Building strong relationships with insurance carriers ensures that agents have the backing and tools they need to serve their clients effectively.

Agents should not overlook the value of **online learning platforms and industry publications.** Websites like LIMRA (Life Insurance and Market Research Association) offer research reports, market analysis, and insights into consumer behavior. Regularly reading industry publications such as *Insurance Newsnet* or *Advisor Today* helps agents stay informed about trends, challenges, and opportunities in the life insurance market. Blogs, podcasts, and YouTube channels hosted by industry leaders also provide practical tips and inspiration for agents looking to refine their strategies and grow their businesses.

For agents aiming to expand their client base, **lead generation platforms** are indispensable. Websites like Policygenius, QuoteWizard, and other online insurance marketplaces connect agents with potential clients actively seeking coverage. While these platforms often come at a cost, they provide a steady stream of qualified leads, saving agents time and effort in prospecting. Pairing these tools with a strong online presence, such as a professional website and active social media profiles, enhances visibility and credibility.

Building a successful life insurance business also requires **financial resources and planning.** Agents should evaluate "where" they can secure funding or allocate resources to grow their operations. This might include investing in marketing campaigns, hiring additional staff, or upgrading office equipment. For newer agents or those running independent practices, exploring small business loans, grants, or partnerships can provide the financial backing needed to scale their business effectively.

Mentorship and peer groups are another vital resource for growth. Connecting with experienced agents who have navigated similar challenges provides guidance, support, and perspective. Peer groups, whether formal or informal, create opportunities for brainstorming, sharing best practices, and holding one another accountable. These relationships can inspire creativity and foster a collaborative environment where agents learn from each other's successes and setbacks.

Lastly, **personal development resources** are often overlooked but equally important. Growing a business requires resilience, confidence, and excellent communication skills. Investing in personal development through books, workshops, or coaching sessions can help agents cultivate the mindset and habits needed for long-term success. For example, reading books on sales psychology or attending workshops on emotional intelligence can enhance an agent's ability to connect with clients and handle objections effectively.

In conclusion, the "where" in growing a life insurance business lies in a combination of professional networks, continuing education, technology, community connections, insurer support, and personal development. By actively seeking out and utilizing these resources, agents can overcome challenges, stay competitive, and build a thriving career. The key is not just identifying these opportunities but also committing to leverage them effectively and consistently for sustained growth.

Section XXVII

When?

Committing Your Time and Energy to Consistent Growth and Improvement

Timing is everything when it comes to achieving success in the life insurance industry. The **when** is not a one-time decision or a fleeting moment—it is an ongoing commitment to dedicate your time and energy consistently toward growth and improvement. In a field where client needs, industry trends, and personal skills must continually evolve, the most successful agents understand that progress is built not on occasional effort, but on sustained dedication.

The first step to embracing the **when** is recognizing that growth requires daily action. Success doesn't happen overnight; it's the result of deliberate, consistent effort over time. Life insurance agents who prioritize continuous improvement embed habits into their daily routines that contribute to long-term achievements. This might include setting aside time each day for prospecting, following up with leads, or refining their product knowledge. For example, dedicating one hour every morning to outreach ensures a steady stream of potential clients, while regularly scheduling time for professional development keeps skills sharp and relevant.

Consistency also means showing up even when challenges arise. The life insurance industry is competitive, and agents often face rejection, changing market conditions, or demanding workloads. Committing your time and energy doesn't mean avoiding these challenges but embracing them as opportunities for growth. For instance, when faced with a difficult objection from a client, an agent who is dedicated to improvement will take the time to reflect, seek advice, or attend training to strengthen their response skills. These small, consistent efforts to address weaknesses build resilience and confidence over time.

Another aspect of **when** is recognizing the importance of time management. Success in the life insurance business requires balancing multiple priorities, including client consultations, administrative tasks, marketing efforts, and personal development. Agents who are intentional about how they spend their time are more likely to achieve their goals. This involves setting clear schedules, prioritizing high-value activities, and eliminating distractions. For example, an agent might designate specific days for client meetings and reserve evenings for studying new industry trends or completing certifications. Structuring your time ensures that every moment contributes meaningfully to growth and improvement.

Commit your time and energy also means being proactive rather than reactive. Waiting for the perfect moment to start something often results in missed opportunities. The best time to improve your skills, deepen your client relationships, or explore new markets is always **NOW**. For instance, if an agent has been considering adopting a new CRM system or launching a digital marketing campaign, delaying these actions only postpones the benefits. By taking initiative and acting in the present, agents can stay ahead of the competition and continually expand their capabilities.

Long-term growth also depends on recognizing the cyclical nature of commitment. There will be seasons of intense effort—such as building a client base or launching a new initiative—and periods of reflection and adjustment. During quieter times, agents should focus on self-assessment and planning. For example, at the end of each year, an agent might review their performance, identify areas for improvement, and set new goals for the coming months. These cycles of action and reflection ensure that growth remains intentional and aligned with overall objectives.

Investing your energy in consistent improvement also requires a commitment to adaptability. The life insurance industry is constantly evolving, with new products, technologies, and regulations shaping the landscape. Agents who dedicate themselves to staying informed and flexible are better equipped to navigate these changes. For example, an agent who consistently learns about digital tools, such as virtual meeting platforms or AI-driven analytics, can enhance client interactions and streamline operations. Adaptability ensures that time and energy are spent effectively, even in uncertain or changing circumstances.

Another dimension of the **when** is *understanding the cumulative power of consistent effort.* Small, incremental improvements may not seem significant in the moment, but over time, they compound into substantial progress. For instance, an agent who commits to reading one article about financial planning each day will, by the end of a year, have gained a wealth of knowledge that sets them apart from competitors. Similarly, dedicating time to build relationships—such as following up with clients regularly or attending networking events—

creates a foundation for long-term trust and growth.

Finally, *committing your time and energy means embracing the idea that improvement is an ongoing journey rather than a destination.* There is always more to learn, new skills to develop, and better ways to serve clients. This mindset fosters a culture of lifelong learning and continuous self-improvement. For example, even experienced agents can benefit from attending advanced training programs, exploring emerging markets, or seeking mentorship from industry leaders. The key is to view every moment as an opportunity to grow, refine your craft, and move closer to your goals.

In conclusion, the **'when'** of growth and improvement in the life insurance industry is not about waiting for the right time but about consistently dedicating your time and energy to the process. By committing to daily actions, managing your time effectively, and embracing a mindset of continuous learning, you position yourself for sustained success. Growth is not achieved in leaps but in steady steps taken with purpose and persistence. The time to act is always now, and the effort you invest today will define the professional you become tomorrow.